*We dedicate this book to Bill Foege,
who has pointed the way to global health equity,
provided a role model in how we might achieve it,
and inspired us and countless others to adopt his
values of social justice, integrity, collaboration,
and optimism.*

REAL COLLABORATION

What It Takes for Global Health to Succeed

Mark L. Rosenberg, Elisabeth S. Hayes,
Margaret H. McIntyre, and Nancy Neill

With a preface by William H. Foege

University of California Press   Berkeley   Los Angeles
Milbank Memorial Fund   New York

The Milbank Memorial Fund is an endowed operating foundation
that engages in nonpartisan analysis, study, research, and
communication on significant issues in health policy. In the
Fund's own publications, in reports, films, or books it publishes
with other organizations, and in articles it commissions for
publication by other organizations, the Fund endeavors to
maintain the highest standards for accuracy and fairness.
Statements by individual authors, however, do not necessarily
reflect opinions or factual determinations of the Fund. For
more information, visit www.milbank.org.

University of California Press, one of the most distinguished
university presses in the United States, enriches lives around the
world by advancing scholarship in the humanities, social sciences,
and natural sciences. Its activities are supported by the UC Press
Foundation and by philanthropic contributions from individuals
and institutions. For more information, visit www.ucpress.edu.

University of California Press
Berkeley and Los Angeles, California

University of California Press, Ltd.
London, England

© 2010 by the Regents of the University of California

Cataloging-in-publication data is on file
with the Library of Congress.

California/Milbank Books on Health and the Public, 20

ISBN-13: 978-0-520-25950-8 (cloth); 978-0-520-25951-5 (paper)

Manufactured in the United States of America

12   11   10   09   08   07   06   05
10   9   8   7   6   5   4   3   2   1

The paper used in this publication meets the minimum
requirements of ANSI/NISO Z39.48-1992 (R 1997) *(Permanence
of Paper).*

CONTENTS

Foreword by Daniel M. Fox, Carmen Hooker Odom, and Samuel L. Milbank   ix

Preface by William H. Foege   xi

Acknowledgments   xv

1. Introduction: Why Collaboration Matters and Why It Happens Too Rarely   1

PART ONE: CHALLENGES AFFECTING COLLABORATION

2. The Diverse Landscape of Global Health   17

3. Nature of the Disease / Threat   31

4. Cultural and Social Challenges   52

PART TWO: INSIGHTS FROM PAST PARTNERSHIPS

5. Lessons along the Partnership Pathway   69

6. The First Mile   85

7. The Journey: Discipline and Flexibility in Management   108

8. The Journey: Complementary Leadership Roles   127

9. The Last Mile   143

10. Ways for Donors to Encourage Collaboration   157

11. Conclusion: The Purpose of Real Collaboration   176

TOOLKITS   The First Mile   179

The Journey: Management   197

The Journey: Leadership   211

The Last Mile   222

The Donor   233

APPENDIX 1. Coalitions and Collaboration in Global Health: A Dialogue Hosted by the Task Force for Global Health (formerly the Task Force for Child Survival and Development)   243

APPENDIX 2. Coalitions and Collaboration in Global Health: A Symposium for Global Health Leaders   245

Works Cited   249

Index   253

Links to writable PDF versions of the Toolkits, as well as to the films, may be found at www.ucpress.edu/9780520259508.

The Milbank Memorial Fund is an endowed operating foundation that works to improve health by helping decision makers in the public and private sectors acquire and use the best available evidence to inform policy for health care and population health. The Fund has engaged in nonpartisan analysis, study, research, and communication about significant issues in health policy about significant issues in health policy since its inception in 1905.

This is the twentieth book of the series of California/Milbank Books on Health and the Public. The publishing partnership between the Fund and the University of California Press encourages the synthesis and communication of findings from research and experience that could contribute to more effective health policy.

In *Real Collaboration: What It Takes for Global Health to Succeed*, the authors, Mark Rosenberg, Elisabeth Hayes, Margaret McIntyre, and Nancy Neill, tackle the question, How can partnerships in global health perform better? The word "collaboration" has many meanings and is often referred to as "cooperation" and "coordination." Using examples of partnerships that have attempted to address particular threats to health, the authors present in rich detail their concept of the four stages of "real" collaboration. They provide a comprehensive, practical construct—the Partnership Pathway—which identifies elements that contribute to success at each stage.

The authors open the first chapter with an example of an extremely successful partnership to address a global health issue and then explore other successful partnerships in subsequent chapters. But they also offer thoughtful analysis, with examples, of why many investments in global health partnerships do not pay off and why many partnerships fall short of their potential.

The authors conducted more than one hundred interviews and held numerous meetings with key thought leaders in the fields of organizational development, education, business, government, and global health. As a result, they "anchor" their "research in the realities of day-to-day work in a partnership."

Throughout the book the authors examine how perceptions of threats to health and the policies to address them have changed since the mid-1980s and identify new challenges ahead. They emphasize that effective collaboration is more important than ever—and more difficult to achieve. As a result of the authors' thorough research and analysis, this book should be useful for policymakers in national and multinational donor organizations, foundations, and nongovernmental service organizations as well as for professionals in global health.

Daniel M. Fox
President Emeritus

Carmen Hooker Odom
President

Samuel L. Milbank
Chairman

A boy leads a blind man, holding onto a stick. It's a familiar and evocative sculpture for those who visit the headquarters of the World Health Organization, the Carter Center, the World Bank, and Merck. I thought of that sculpture recently when I started using a cane because of a fracture. My two-year-old granddaughter sometimes walked with me, and she held onto the cane and limped also. I realized she was showing empathy. She had inherited from her parents the idea that you should treat each other respectfully and empathetically, as the boy does in the sculpture. What a good symbol that sculpture is for global health in the twenty-first century. It demonstrates the dependency we have on each other, and it demonstrates collaborative intent. One human reaching out to help another.

We have never been in a better position to extend a hand to people around the globe. With the resources of United Nations agencies; the foundations endowed by Rockefeller, Gates, Buffet, and Turner; Rotary International; pharmaceutical companies; bilaterals; multilaterals; and thousands of nongovernmental organizations, we have an abundance to tap that is beyond anything we could have imagined fifty years ago. And the most important lesson of those fifty years is that collaboration is the best way to make those resources count. Real collaboration. The give-and-take of human beings who are so dedicated to a mission they will set aside the politics of organizations, share the difficulties, and invent solutions together.

What can we do to make that kind of collaboration more common in global health? Part of the answer lies in the spirit we bring to our work—the empathetic and respectful spirit of that young boy holding the stick. But another part lies in the brave responsibility he shows. We can demonstrate both aspects by taking collaboration seriously as a discipline and applying it in our work through concrete actions. We can start by sharing the lessons learned from past collaborations. Winston Churchill once said, "Play the game for more than you can afford to lose, only then will you learn the game." That's where we are today. With the scale of assets now going into global health, we are betting more than we can afford to lose, and we simply have to learn the rules of this game. This book is a starting point because it captures many of those "rules" or lessons in the words of those who have learned them in the villages of developing countries. We need to make those lessons widely accessible and encourage people to use them in developing course curricula, program plans, and evaluations. As we do, we can create a shared understanding across global health of what makes a partnership successful. We will know the rules for how to win this game.

We should also begin to cultivate the leadership skills needed for collaboration. These are not the traditional leadership skills. Collaboration requires leadership through persuasion and relationship building because the real coalition skills are interpersonal. As the stories told throughout this book show, this kind of leadership is not about making and imposing smart decisions but about surfacing ideas, facilitating thoughtful discussions, listening to different perspectives, handling conflict, and voicing consensus as it develops. It conveys empathy and respect for our fellow human beings and requires that we suppress our own egos.

Global health leaders also need to come together and agree on the most critical priorities and how to address them. What are the twenty big areas we should be focusing on? Incredibly, we have no answer to that question today because no single agency or foundation plays a central leadership role. Across global health we lack coordination in tackling major diseases and threats, such as HIV/AIDS. So we squander resources by duplicating efforts or leaving gaps in the populations we serve, and millions suffer and die needlessly. To prevent this misery, we need to join forces and agree on our top global health priorities and how we will organize to tackle them. Chapter 10 suggests a forum for that kind of discussion.

And, finally, we need to find a means of holding UN agencies and large donors accountable for their stated missions. These missions invariably require collaboration, but it's so easy for large agencies or foundations to become arrogant about what they're doing. When they do, they fail to do the central thing that would allow them to succeed: to really collaborate, to learn from the people they're trying to help and to learn from their partners. We need to find a way to hold them accountable for their failures to collaborate. If we monitored those agencies and donors against their missions, it would motivate them to take a fresh look at what they're doing.

Now I'll come back to the image of that young boy leading the blind man and the inspiring sense of responsibility and respect he embodies. The responsibility for taking these actions falls on the shoulders of a relatively small group, and if you're reading this book, you are in that group. As we take these steps to build the discipline of collaboration into our work, we also need to show respect for our partners from the developing world, from government, from NGOs, or from the private sector. They are the ones who can teach us how to move forward. Medical knowledge is not enough. Western leadership is not enough. Money is not enough. We must depend on each other. Only with respect for what all of us can contribute will we understand the best way to approach global health threats. Only then can we use the abundant resources available in a way that opens up the possibility of global health equity in the twenty-first century.

William H. Foege

ACKNOWLEDGMENTS

Our greatest debt is to Dr. William H. Foege, who gave us our earliest insights into what it takes to achieve real collaboration. He gave unstintingly of his time, introduced us to key players on the international scene, and was a continuous source of both learning and inspiration.

While working on this book, we've encountered a remarkably enthusiastic response from many other global health leaders, donor representatives, health agencies, and individuals who responded to our numerous phone calls, interviews, and meeting requests. The subject is clearly important to them, and they shared with us a wealth of information, insights, and constructive feedback. Their responses led to an understanding of the dynamics of individual partnerships and the evolution of all the combined efforts to address individual diseases and health threats. We've laid out that understanding in these pages. Some of these people joined our advisory group, giving generously of their time and experience to help us shape the direction of our research. Others participated in the Global Health Leadership Symposium at the Carter Center in 2006, speaking out about the things global health needs to do to become more collaborative. These discussions helped us refine the frameworks included in this book. (See appendixes 1 and 2 for a list of participants at each event.) President Jimmy Carter energized all of us with a spontaneous commitment to support further work on collaboration. One result was the formation of the Center for Global Health Collaboration, based at the Task Force for Global Health, formerly the Task Force for Child Survival and Development in Atlanta.

The members of the Atlanta Coalition for Global Health—CARE, the Centers for Disease Control and Prevention (CDC), the CDC Foundation, the Morehouse School of Medicine, the Rollins School of Public Health, and the Task Force for Child Survival and Development—supported our early efforts and the Carter Center symposium in 2006.

A third event in the life of this research and book project was a meeting of the Review Committee in 2008. The committee took the time to read and critique an earlier draft of this book, and their enthusiasm and tough questions stimulated us to think harder and learn more. Participating in the committee were Seth Berkley, Heidi Bresnahan, Alison Drayton, Dan Fox, Larry Gostin, Srishti Gupta, Clarion Johnson, Jordan Kassalow, Jacob Kumaresan, Adetokunbo Lucas, Carmen Hooker Odom, Ian Smith, Pascal Villeneuve, Lynne Withey, and Ray Yip. We are very appreciative of the many ways in which these individuals helped to improve this work.

Several deans of schools of public health also helped us understand the best way to teach collaboration skills to future generations of public health leaders. We want to thank Barry Bloom, Mushtaque Chowdhury, Jim Curran, Andy Haines, Michael Klag, Allan Rosenfield, and Harrison Spencer.

Individuals from our three funders were involved in our research, and many of them also participated in the key events mentioned earlier. In particular, we would like to thank Sally Stansfield and Kathy Cahill from the Bill & Melinda Gates Foundation; George Brown, Derek Yach, and Ariel Pablos-Mendez from the Rockefeller Foundation; and Bill Gimson, Stephen Blount, and Chad Martin from the CDC.

Our publishers and film crew also nurtured our efforts. We would like to thank Dan Fox, Carmen Hooker Odom, and Heidi Bresnahan from the Milbank Memorial Fund and Lynne Withey from the University of California Press. Without their support this book and the companion film would not have been possible. In addition, we owe special appreciation to several people from Richard Stanley Productions for producing the film: Richard Stanley for his engaging interviews with key leaders in global health, Matt Stanley for his editing, and Kerry Meyer and Hugh Hood for their excellent filming.

Some other individuals deserve special recognition: Ian Smith from WHO, who provided unfailing support throughout the life of this project and gave us the opportunity to hold a key workshop with WHO directors involved in partnerships; Srishti Gupta of McKinsey & Company, who shared her thoughtful analysis and perspectives on governance and global health partnerships; James Austin of the Harvard Business School, who helped to facilitate the Carter Center Symposium and shared his insights into business and nonprofit partnerships; Rick Gilkey of Emory University Goizueta Business School, who reviewed the Toolkits that accompany this book and provided guidance on the key elements of leadership; Alan Slobodnik and Louis de Merode, who shared with us their guidance on organizational cultures and teams; and Lou Rowitz, who helped us understand the complexities of training people in leadership. Contributors also included interns and staff members at the Task Force for Global Health who helped in researching the concepts, health threats, and information related to the Toolkits: JulieMarie Goupil, Lauren Giles, Liz Cannella, Soobin Parks, Meaghan House, Alyssa Davis, and Rebecca Willis. Finally, we would like to thank Carter Cowden for her help preparing the manuscript for publication.

A book like this, based on dozens of individual stories, is dependent on the participation of so many people. We are grateful to all of them for their honesty and generosity in shaping this perspective on real collaboration.

Chapter 1 | INTRODUCTION

Why Collaboration Matters and
Why It Happens Too Rarely

In the mid-1980s several organizations involved in global health wrestled with how to get a stalled immunization effort back on track. They formed the Task Force for Child Survival, a partnership that quickly reinvigorated the effort and allowed the organizations to reach the goal.[1] The partnership had another impact: it provided a stunning example of what partnerships could achieve through real collaboration. Briefly, this is how the story of the Task Force unfolded.

In 1974 member states of the World Health Organization (WHO) had passed a resolution to bring vaccines to children across the globe. At the Alma Ata Conference in 1978 they had set a concrete goal of immunizing 80 percent of the world's children against common childhood diseases by 1990. But by 1984, after climbing from 5 percent to 20 percent, immunization coverage had leveled off.

To break the impasse, these organizations decided to form a task force composed of senior leaders from WHO, the United Nations Development Program (UNDP), the World Bank, UNICEF, and the Rockefeller Foundation. They formed a secretariat, the Task Force for Child Survival, and charged it with helping the partnership rejuvenate immunization efforts and overcome the competitive and divisive forces that had slowed down the previous effort. The Task Force did more than coordinate efforts of the respective organizations. The individuals in the partnership were able to look beyond the separate interests of their own organizations and problem-solve together. They became a team. Under their guidance the Task Force secretariat created a unified plan of action, addressed political roadblocks to pave the way for in-country efforts, solved technical problems as they arose, and kept the commitment and momentum alive.

By 1990 this partnership had raised immunization rates from 20 percent to 80 percent. James Grant, director of UNICEF at the time, called the initiative the "largest peacetime mobilization in the history of the earth."[2]

This collaboration would become a touchstone in global health.

Because of efforts like this, the closing decade of the twentieth century saw a rapid rise in partnerships responding to emerging health threats. From 1995 to 2000, for example, key partnerships (including "alliances" and "coalitions") emerged in the following five disease and threat areas:

- *Onchocerciasis (1995)*. The African Program for Onchocerciasis Control (APOC) launched an effort to help local communities in nineteen African countries organize and manage treatment for river blindness with the drug Mectizan. APOC was formed by the World Bank, WHO, UNDP, the Food and Agriculture Organization of the United Nations (FAO), the governments of nineteen developing countries and twenty-seven donor countries, twenty nongovernmental organizations (NGOs), and the global pharmaceutical Merck.
- *HIV/AIDS (1996)*. Seven UN agencies established the joint United Nations program called UNAIDS.
- *Tuberculosis (1998)*. Attendees at the World Conference on Lung Health launched the STOP-TB initiative.
- *Malaria (1998)*. WHO, UNICEF, UNDP, the World Bank, and other partners founded the Roll Back Malaria Partnership (RBM), with the goal of cutting the incidence of malaria in half by 2010.
- *Vaccine preventable diseases (1999)*. A combination of governments, foundations, development agencies, and NGOs formed the Global Alliance for Vaccines and Immunization (GAVI).

Partnerships had become the preferred approach to global health.

As the coordination costs of global partnerships became clearer, however, participants and donors had second thoughts. Participants themselves became more conscious of the huge time requirement for traveling to global meetings and the slow pace of building trust across organizations, time zones, and cultures. Donors began looking at the return they were getting on their investment of time, effort, and money, to see if partnerships really paid off.

KEY DONOR REPORTS: DO PARTNERSHIPS PAY OFF?

The attempt to measure impact was complicated. While businesses typically measure cost-effectiveness, public health had traditionally measured input or output—the level of demand for services or the number of people treated, for example. Russell Linden, a writer and lecturer on management, recalls: "When I directed a nonprofit organization that served handicapped people and their families back in the 1970s, I simply had to show an increasing demand for my nonprofit's programs in order to justify a budget increase from its funding agencies."[3]

By the 1990s, however, that approach to measurement was no longer considered satisfactory, and funders began to look for better ways to measure results (reduction in the number of people affected by a disease, for instance) and, ultimately, cost-effectiveness. Measuring such impacts was challenging, since global health projects typically lacked the accountability, tracking systems, and financial controls common in business. Nevertheless, two donors analyzed the results of projects they had funded, and produced reports: The Bill & Melinda Gates Foundation (the Gates Foundation) and the British government's Department for International Development (DFID).

The Gates report, developed by a team from the management consulting firm McKinsey & Company and released in April 2002, recognized the dominant role partnerships had come to play in global health: "Simply put, there are few global public health challenges where any single player has the funding, research, and delivery capabilities required to solve the problem on a worldwide scale. . . . As one measure of their importance, alliances represent nearly 80 percent of the value of global health investments made by the Bill & Melinda Gates Foundation."[4] The McKinsey team found that "more than 80 percent of public health alliances appear to be working."[5] By "working," they meant the alliance had accelerated, improved, or reduced the cost of an initiative, compared with what agencies could have done on their own. But using a higher standard for realizing their potential, the Gates report concluded that those alliances had not performed as well: "For example, some alliances spend the first six to eighteen months doing little more than developing operating plans rather than attacking the disease burden. And other alliances, even after being launched, are hamstrung by limited resources or difficulties in arriving at decisions among the various partner organizations."[6] Partnerships, in other words, were worthwhile, but many were underperforming.

DFID reached a similar conclusion in its report, released in 2004. It looked at the global health partnerships (GHPs) it had been involved in and concluded that "individual GHPs are seen overall as having a positive impact in terms both of achieving their own objectives and of being welcomed by countries studied.... The general theme of findings from most evaluations is one of GHP success, but with clear scope for yet further achievement if challenges are resolved."[7] The return-on-investment answer was a qualified yes. Even in the polite language of the reports, it was clear many of these partnerships fell far short of their potential. An improvement opportunity undoubtedly existed.

LINK BETWEEN SUCCESS AND CLOSE COLLABORATION

How could partnerships perform better? As these reports were being released, we had already begun to explore the issue of how to improve ,

> "How is it possible that in the year 2006 we can be losing so many young women unnecessarily? We have the drugs to keep them alive. How is this possible? And you know that it's happening because of the failure, the failure of the world at the level of the country, to join together and respond to the pandemic, to defeat it, to collaborate with each other in the service of keeping these women alive so that the orphans aren't left behind, so these young women have a life to lead, and it's not snuffed out in agony."
>
> STEPHEN LEWIS, United Nations special envoy for HIV/AIDS in Africa, upon returning from a women's HIV/AIDS ward in Mozambique, October 19, 2006, interview

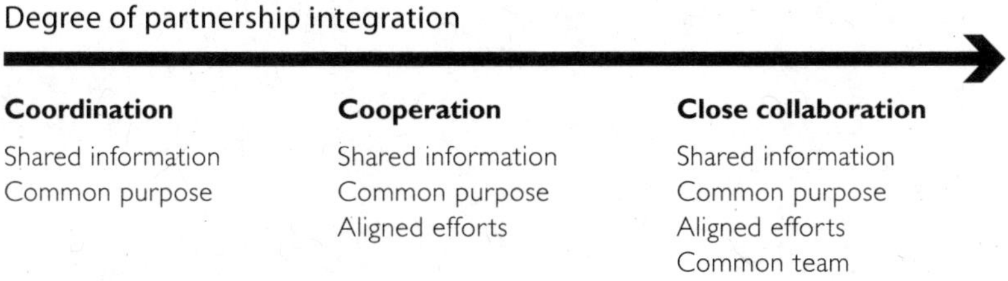

Degree of partnership integration

→

Coordination	Cooperation	Close collaboration
Shared information	Shared information	Shared information
Common purpose	Common purpose	Common purpose
	Aligned efforts	Aligned efforts
		Common team

FIGURE 1.1   The spectrum of collaboration. **Partnerships exist along a spectrum from coordination, to cooperation, to close collaboration.**

collaboration in global health. To begin with, we found that no definition of collaboration was widely accepted. Global health leaders (from all sectors) use the word "collaboration" broadly. As Linden points out, "To some, it suggests polite cooperation. To others, it includes everything from shared data to joint operations."[8] We realized that collaborative partnerships existed along a spectrum, from having a common purpose but *operating independently* (perhaps with one organization coordinating activities) to aligning efforts and *acting cooperatively* to actually *forming an integrated team,* where members work together toward a single shared goal. The words "coordination," "cooperation," and "close collaboration" are sometimes used to make distinctions along that spectrum and suggest a useful framework.

Using this spectrum (Figure 1.1 and Table 1.1), we looked for examples of each type of collaboration in global health, and we began to understand some distinctions. The left side—coordinating in some way but continuing to operate independently—seems to be the most feasible way to respond to such large disasters as the tsunami that struck Indonesia in 2004 and Hurricane Katrina, which ravaged the Gulf Coast of the United States in 2005. For the tsunami UN officials played a major role in coordinating efforts. These efforts were run in parallel, without much sharing of information about survivors' needs and capabilities. A report from the Federation of the Red Cross and Red Crescent Societies indicates that fewer than a quarter of the two hundred agencies present in Aceh a month after the tsunami had provided UN coordinators with activity reports.[9] While more extensive sharing of information would undoubtedly have

TABLE 1.1 Coordination, cooperation, collaboration

Coordination is appropriate when	Cooperation is appropriate when	Close collaboration is appropriate when
A recognized authority is available to coordinate efforts	The sharing of information will allow participants to accomplish a goal they cannot reach through parallel efforts	The timeframe is measured in years, not months
Implementation is limited to a single country or region		The goal is so ambitious, it cannot be met through coordination or cooperation
An immediate and efficient response is required (as with disasters)		The nature of disease/threat presents formidable social and political challenges
		A core team of willing members emerges, willing to invest time and expertise

been helpful, organizations will always be driven to saves lives first in times of disaster.

The middle of the spectrum—acting cooperatively—allows a more coordinated and targeted response. Clinton Foundation efforts to support developing nations are a good example. After conducting focus groups in Africa to determine the key development issue, the foundation heard a clear answer: AIDS! With treatment then averaging US$320 per case each year, the cost of drugs was a major problem, and analysis showed that unpredictable demand kept prices high. The foundation pooled demand from twelve countries, ensuring predictability of demand so that drug companies could manage production and lower costs. Interestingly, no drugs were ordered through the foundation: orders and shipments went directly between countries and drug companies. The Clinton Foundation simply helped these countries cooperate to effectively share information as a way to lower costs.

The right side of the spectrum—forming an integrated team—is appropriate, we realized, in highly challenging, long-term projects like the childhood immunization project of the 1980s. Because the Task Force for Child Survival became an integrated team, they were able to debate challenges and come up with practical solutions. This close form of collaboration, referred to in the title of this book as "real collaboration," is not and should not be the norm for global health partnerships, because it requires the greatest resources. It is also, however, absolutely necessary to accomplish certain goals and is the most powerful form of collaboration.

Rob Lehman, who heads the Fetzer Institute, describes the nature of close collaboration. "Collaboration, on the surface, is about bringing together resources, both financial and intellectual, to work toward a common purpose. But true collaboration has an 'inside,' a deeper more radical meaning." He continues: "The inner life of collaboration is about states of mind and spirit that are open—open to self-examination, open to growth, open to trust, and open to mutual action. . . . The practices of true collaboration are those practices of awareness, listening, and speaking that bring us into openness and receptivity."[10] After interviewing dozens of global health leaders throughout the course of our research, we are convinced this willingness of partners to set aside business-as-usual and consider new possibilities together is what sets apart the most successful collaborations.

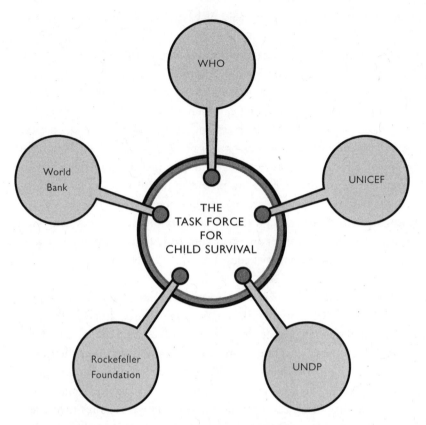

FIGURE 1.2   The Task Force for Child Survival. **Close collaboration takes place between individuals, not between the organizations they represent.**

As with the Task Force for Child Survival, close collaboration has to take place between the individuals in the partnership, not between the organizations they represent. Open, productive debates and problem solving can only occur among a core team of individuals who bring the passion, willingness to understand other points of view, creativity, and sheer force of will to make the effort work. In Figure 1.2 these individuals are indicated inside the center circle. This realization helped us define what our book would not be about (Table 1.2). After considering the spectrum of collaboration, we realized we had found an area of focus for our research: partnerships pursuing a single, shared goal performed better when they became an integrated

TABLE 1.2 This book is not

A survey of all global health partnerships
An exploration of partnerships that
· lack a core team of individuals working together over time
· involve constantly rotating representatives of member agencies
· rely on presentations as the primary form of communication
· are semipermanent, comprised of individuals whose primary identification
  is with the partnership itself
An academic review with extensive technical references, facts, and footnotes

team—the end of the spectrum called "close collaboration." That was where we wanted to concentrate our research efforts.

RESEARCH ON CLOSE COLLABORATION

Unfortunately, that kind of collaboration does not happen often. Leaders in the field of global health often talk about "collaboration" as if it were an ordinary and expected quality of partnerships. And it is, if you consider the spectrum of definitions. However, our experiences at the Task Force for Global Health (the Task Force) have taught us that, despite excellent role models and our predisposition to work collaboratively, our own teams and our colleagues' teams often lack the insights and skills to achieve real collaboration. At the Task Force, for example, we had ample opportunity to work collaboratively. Tackling global issues like tuberculosis, river blindness, and the rising toll of road-traffic injuries in developing countries meant we had the chance to work with partners across the world, including governments, UN agencies, and NGOs. But these partnerships often failed to deliver the full impact we had anticipated. Why was that? And what could we do about it?

In 2004, with grants from the Gates Foundation, the Rockefeller Foundation, and the Centers for Disease Control, we launched a research effort to explore the question, How can global health leaders achieve close collaboration and have a bigger impact? When our planning was complete, we had decided to conduct more than a hundred interviews, hold dozens of face-to-face meetings with thought leaders in the fields of collaboration and global health, form an advisory group to provide early guidance, and convene a symposium to communicate and explore our emerging conclusions. We would look for specific examples of partnerships that either achieved close collaboration or learned valuable lessons through their successes and failures. And we would consider each partnership in the broad context of other efforts to address the disease/threat, outlining the history of those efforts.

The most important part of our research turned out to be the interviews. People from global health, organizational development, education, business, and government were candid and engaging, working with us to make sense of the contradictions and challenges inherent in every global health project. They also told us the stories that anchored our research in the realities of day-to-day work in a partnership.

Based on their input, we came up with a list of partnerships that demonstrated the elements needed for close collaboration (Table 1.3). Bill Foege, former director of the CDC and a leader in numerous global health partnerships, provided a great deal of guidance in making these selections, encouraging us to include such partnerships as the bottom three in the table, which are focused on political outcomes and are inherently more difficult to measure. We did not select the partnerships based on their success or because they represented the full range of global health issues. Rather, we chose them because they were rich in lessons to apply to other partnerships and because the partners were willing to look back on their efforts to reflect on their strengths and weaknesses. We have supplemented this list with lessons from efforts to address other diseases, such as HIV/AIDS, malaria, and guinea worm.

These were not broad efforts to attack a disease/threat, and they were not permanent organizations. They were temporary partnerships of people whose primary identifications were with their own organizations.[11] While each of these partnerships had their imperfections, the stories are about real collaboration—those *rare* times when people from different organizations come together with passion and purpose and accomplish dramatically more than any agency or person could do alone. After almost two years of research, we convened an advisory group in November 2005 to help us calibrate what we had learned. With their input over the next year we refined the framework for organizing the lessons learned and began drafting this book.

TABLE 1.3 Example cases

Disease/threat	Partnership	Type	Impact
Smallpox	Partnership to eliminate smallpox in India (1973–1975)	Intervention	Eradicated smallpox in India
Childhood immunization	Task Force for Child Survival (1984–1990)	Intervention	Achieved goal of immunizing 80 percent of the world's children
Polio	Polio partnership of the Americas (1985–1991)	Intervention	Eradicated polio in the Americas
River blindness (onchocerciasis)	African Programme for Onchocerciasis Control (since 1995)	Intervention	By 2006, 117,000 communities were conducting their own treatment programs for more than 46 million people.
Tobacco	Policy Advisory Committee of the Tobacco Free Initiative (1999–2003)	Advocacy to generate political will	Led to adoption by the WHA of a Framework Convention that focused on advertising, air quality controls, and smuggling
Road-traffic injuries	Global Road Safety Steering Committee (2002–2004)	Advocacy to generate political will	Resulted in a UN General Assembly meeting and resolution calling for international cooperation to deal with road safety in developing countries
TB	PARTNERS TB Control Program (2000–2006)	Pilot program to prove feasibility of integrating TB and MDR-TB treatment	Demonstrated feasibility of treating MDR-TB and led to a declaration by WHO that MDR-TB should be treated wherever it occurs

In October 2006 more than a hundred leaders from the public, private, and social sectors joined us for a symposium at the Carter Center, called "Coalitions and Collaboration in Global Health." Former president Jimmy Carter challenged us to generate concrete proposals for improving collaboration; Bill Foege called for a passionate commitment to making real collaboration a priority; and leaders from every sector spoke honestly about the shortfalls of projects, suggesting ideas for better collaboration.

Susan Holck, director of general management with WHO, was one of those leaders. We had invited Holck to participate in a panel, drawing on her experience in the development of UNAIDS. She told us this story:

> Before coming to the symposium a colleague had asked her, referring to the early days of UNAIDS, "Are you going to tell the truth?" Her response: "Of course, there's no reason not to tell the story now, ten years later."
>
> According to Holck, the early problem of UNAIDS "was a failure of the global health community to recognize the extent of the problem and really work together to do something about it. . . . There were conflicting goals among the specific organizations involved, WHO, UNICEF, World Bank, and UNDP in particular. . . . Conflicting goals of the individuals involved . . . and the fear of loss of power. I think that played an enormous role, that the individuals who were in a position of power in the early days of AIDS, before UNAIDS was born, feared loss of power. . . . The donors effectively forced this collaboration on the UN institutions . . . to set an example in UN reform. Almost no one, in setting up UNAIDS, really had AIDS in mind as the goal for what we were doing."
>
> She added, "Over the years [UNAIDS] did manage to create a central focus. . . . It forced the players to work together."[12]

In honest appraisals like this one, global health leaders shared with us the missteps as well as the successes in their own efforts. In this book we present the assessments in their own voices.

CONCLUSIONS

Repeatedly, during our interviews, we heard the lesson that success in reaching a shared goal comes through close collaboration. Partnerships have the best chance for achieving that when they lay the foundations for collaboration in the First Mile and carry a spirit of shared responsibility along the Journey. Three conclusions support this theme:

1. *Real collaboration is highly challenging because of the complex forces at play in global health efforts.* One of the greatest challenges outside the partnership is the landscape of global health today, a changing web of relationships and expectations. The nature of the disease or threat also presents its own special problems, including social stigmas or political sensitivities. And the cultural and social dynamics within a partnership are particularly challenging in global health, where the diversity of cultures is very broad.

2. *At each stage of a partnership's pathway—the First Mile, the Journey, and the Last Mile—partners need to focus on key tasks and shared responsibilities.* For example, the seeds of success or failure are sown in the early stage of a partnership—that awkward period when disparate organizations come together to start a common effort. Many partnerships begin with a lengthy legal process of chartering (defining roles and processes). These are important activities, but focusing primarily on these processes can make teams miss some of the essential work that needs to be done. The attention in the First Mile should be on gathering the right members, developing a goal that is really shared, and agreeing on the basics of strategy, structure, and roles. By discussing these subjects in a thoughtful, open, and respectful atmosphere, partners can begin to establish the social capital and trust that will carry them through the Journey.

3. *Donors can play an important role by encouraging collaborative practices.* For instance, while the Gates report cited excessive planning by some coalitions, the opposite is just as worrisome. The lack of funding and other assistance to allow for appropriate discussions, relationship building, and planning in the First Mile actually undermines collaboration because projects march on while participants have varying interpretations of what they should be doing. By changing grant requirements to support good collaborative practices (including but not limited to planning), donors can leverage the contribution they make to global health.

The book is divided into two sections that expand on these conclusions: Part 1, challenges affecting collaboration, and Part 2, insights from successful and unsuccessful partnerships. Each chapter draws from the rich stories of those who have provided leadership in global health initiatives. By tapping these findings from people across all sectors, leaders in global health can generate new energy and impetus in global health efforts. If even half of the partnerships appropriate for close collaboration could actually achieve it, the collective impact would mean a sea change in health across the globe. In the remaining partnerships, where close collaboration is inappropriate or the barriers are too high, partners can still find ideas to improve the impact and satisfaction of their work. This book offers the lessons we have learned in the hope these things might happen.

NOTES

1. Although the authors of this book are proud to be associated by name with that partnership, we should clarify that we were not associated with the Task Force for Child Survival in its formative years. We should also note that its successor, the Task Force for Child Survival and Development, has recently changed its name to the Task Force for Global Health.
2. Jim Yong Kim, "William H. Foege—Physician: A Lifelong Battle against Disease," *US News and World Report,* posted November 12, 2007, available online at http://www.usnews.com/articles/news/best-leaders/2007/11/12/william-h-foege.html.
3. Linden, *Working Across Boundaries,* 16.
4. Bill & Melinda Gates Foundation, *Developing Successful Global Health Alliances,* 1.
5. Ibid., 1.
6. Ibid., 2.
7. Caines, *Assessing the Impact of Global Health Partnerships,* 4.
8. Linden, *Working Across Boundaries,* 6.
9. International Federation of Red Cross and Red Crescent Societies, *World Disasters Report 2005,* Chapter 1.
10. Lehman as quoted in Olson and Harris, "Defining Common Work," 6.
11. In chapter 3 we look at broader efforts to lay a context for individual partnerships.
12. Holck's presentation at Coalitions and Collaboration in Global Health: A Symposium for Global Health Leaders, October 19, 2006.

PART I | CHALLENGES AFFECTING COLLABORATION

When we started the research for this book, we were keenly aware of some of the changing dynamics in global health. More diverse players were now at the table when a coalition convened, for example, and many more donors were supporting global health efforts. But how, exactly, did these changes affect collaboration? What could they tell us about practical approaches needed to turn a partnership into an integrated team? We decided to dive into the subject and find how these changing dynamics affected partnerships.

It was an eye-opener for the entire team. The challenges to collaboration were far greater than we had anticipated. The landscape of players and how they related to each other had totally changed. Roles had become unclear, authority had been dispersed, and organizations that wanted to contribute their expertise had no clear place to turn for direction. When it came to the nature of a particular health threat, that too had become more complex than in the past as partnerships dealt with drug resistance and began to incorporate such threats as tobacco and road-traffic injuries into the public health arena. The cultural and social dynamics had also become more challenging as coalitions encountered greater diversity in membership. No wonder partnerships often failed to reach their potential.

Chapters 2, 3, and 4 examine these challenges. We start by taking a broad look at the landscape of global health. We then narrow the focus to look at the technical, social, and political dynamics particular to any one disease or health threat. And finally, we examine ground zero—the social dynamics within a partnership.

Chapter 2 | THE DIVERSE LANDSCAPE OF GLOBAL HEALTH

In 2003 two of our authors, Mark Rosenberg and Margaret McIntyre, experienced firsthand the impact external forces can have on a partnership. They were working on a drug-resistant TB effort in Peru with the Partnership Against Resistant Tuberculosis: A Network for Equity and Resource Sharing (PARTNERS) TB Control Program.[1] Rosenberg recounts the effort:

> It was a very compelling project—showing the feasibility of scaling up the treatment of multi-drug-resistant TB (MDR-TB) to all of Peru and creating an approach to be used across the world. We had great resources: Partners in Health initially supplied the medical staff, Socios en Salud provided on-the-ground management, WHO supplied political and policy expertise, Peru's ministry of health (MINSA) represented the government and provided the local infrastructure for implementation, and the Task Force took on the role of coordinating coalition efforts, helping to promote collaboration among the partners. We were all really excited about the combination of resources we were applying to this problem.
>
> And of course there were the patients. You'd have to be made of steel not to be moved by the victims of this disease and their families. A woman who had lost four grown children to MDR-TB in two years was back at a clinic and under treatment herself. A child who had lost both parents was

coming to a clinic for treatment. We knew we had the potential to prevent tragedy for hundreds if not thousands of TB patients in this country.

We were also committed to helping MINSA develop a strategy for sustainability so they could take the effort forward when we were gone. We knew their task would not be easy at a time when the country was in the midst of continuous political change, replacing people in key positions at MINSA every few months.

One day in the spring of 2003 we were told that almost the entire ministry was being restructured. Health sector reform—with its shift from a disease-specific focus to a primary-care orientation—had reached Peru. We had been hearing about the possibility for months, but we didn't know what it would entail or when it would affect the national TB program (NTP). Suddenly it was a fact: the processes for procuring critical drugs, forming treatment teams, establishing policy, and even distributing supplies were completely disrupted, causing health centers to run out of the most basic supplies.

We worked closely with MINSA to try to get the effort operational again, but it was a long, tedious process. An undercurrent of uncertainty ran through every discussion. How could the NTP staff plan when they didn't know whether they would have a job on Monday morning?

The project ended two years later, and it was a huge success by most measures. The coalition had proven the effectiveness of the treatment; the country had health workers in several areas who were trained to provide the treatment; and we had transferred lessons from Peru to a related PARTNERS project in Tomsk, Russia, proving the approach was feasible in other settings. Most important, the coalition had helped (in conjunction with other projects outside PARTNERS) to change TB policy. In May 2005, WHO announced a global policy change for integrating treatment of drug-susceptible TB and drug-resistant TB: they would now urge every country to provide appropriate treatment for both kinds of TB to anyone who needed it, whether in a rich or poor country.

Not a bad set of results. But we could have done more if we had been better prepared to deal with the global forces affecting public health—in this case, health sector reform. The reform clearly carried benefits. But it also created challenges for our partnership. Under the reform, MINSA no longer had national program managers responsible for a particular disease, such as TB; they were responsible for all health needs in their geographic areas. The country lost the advantage of a team of experienced and committed advocates for treating TB, and global agencies found it exceedingly difficult to find someone who wore a "TB hat" and had the power and understanding needed to help spread the treatment protocol across the country. At best, the rollout of treatment across the country would be delayed. Many victims would die in the meantime.

Rosenberg's comment that "we could have done more" captures the sense of lost opportunity following so many efforts in global health that are conducted amid disruptive changes.

To understand such issues better, we decided to explore how the landscape of individuals and organizations has changed since the mid-1980s. As we did so, we began to see more clearly why partnerships have rapidly increased in global health and why collaboration is top-of-mind for so many leaders in the field. Our research uncovered the following three conclusions:

1. Worldwide public health trends have generated new expectations in global health.
2. The architecture of global health institutions has fragmented into a confusing, ad hoc network of policy shapers and decision makers.
3. As a result, collaboration is more important yet more difficult to achieve.

This chapter presents the support for the first two of these conclusions and draws from them the implications for collaboration, our third point.

NEW EXPECTATIONS IN GLOBAL HEALTH

From a midcentury era of highly limited resources and limited participation in decision making, global health has evolved since the mid-1980s to become a field with far more resources globally, greater attention to public health in developing countries, health services that are integrating prevention and treatment, and increased participation of local citizens. The change has been so fundamental that a new set of expectations prevails today (Figure 2.1).

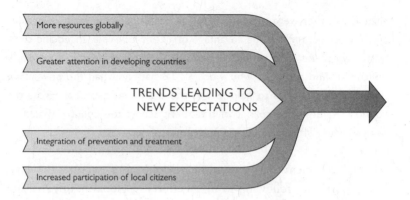

More resources globally

Greater attention in developing countries

TRENDS LEADING TO
NEW EXPECTATIONS

Integration of prevention and treatment

Increased participation of local citizens

FIGURE 2.1   Trends leading to new expectations. **Major trends in global
health have led to greater expectations.**

More Resources Globally

As Bill Foege, senior adviser to the Bill & Melinda Gates Foundation,
commented in the preface to *Global Health Leadership and Management*
in 2005, "Global health has always been compromised by institutional-
ized poverty. Inadequate resources will forever be a concern for global
health workers, but a marked difference has been apparent in the past
two decades."[2] The net resources committed to global health swelled as
the number of NGOs and philanthropies multiplied, pharmaceuticals and
other business organizations became involved, public–private partnerships
became more common (particularly in the product development arena),
and World Bank spending on global health ballooned from US $2 million
in 1970 to US $855 million by 1990. Funds have continued to rise, as a 2007
World Bank report indicates (Figure 2.2).[3]

Investment in technology and cross-border communications to tackle
global disease and manage health crises also rose dramatically with the onset
of AIDS, the avian flu, and major natural disasters (such as earthquakes and
drought). The number of victims of poverty and disease continued to increase,
but these people had the best chance in history of receiving medical help.

Greater Attention in Developing Countries

With the dramatic rise in recent years in resources committed to global
health issues, the attention to public health has also increased in developing countries. For example, health spending has increased substantially in

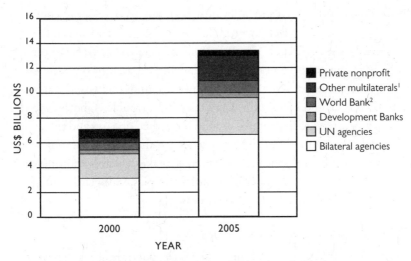

NOTE: This chart includes the latest information available at time of publication.

1. The category of "other mulitlateral" includes the European Union, the Global Alliance for Vaccines and Immunization (GAVI) and the Global Fund to Fight AIDS, Tuberculosis, and Malaria (GFATM).

2. The World Bank total includes only International Development Assistance lending.

FIGURE 2.2   Development assistance for health, by source, 2000–2005. **Net resources committed to global health grew rapidly as more organizations became involved.**

recipient countries since the early 1990s (Table 2.1). Ministers of health and health policymakers have gained greater influence as health has become more closely linked to development issues.

Integration of Prevention and Treatment

While resources were generally increasing and the profile of public health was rising, responsibility for any single disease/threat was being diffused in many developing countries as health sector reform spurred integration of prevention and treatment across diseases/threats.

In many ways health sector reform makes eminent good sense. If it is well executed, it means that many more people receive basic medical help, both preventive care and treatment.

Short-term, however, it has also caused a worrisome misalignment between the integrated public health programs of developing countries and the disease-focused efforts of global health agencies and NGOs that are trying to assist those countries. Participants in global health have been left with an exquisite horizontal-vertical balancing act, and the outcome is still being played out. At first glance the solution sounds obvious: the agencies and NGOs should realign their approach. The trouble is, both expertise and funding tend to be centered around individual diseases and threats. So although a horizontal "health for all" approach aims at collaboration across sectors and programs within a country, it makes collaboration between individual countries and the NGOs, philanthropies, and agencies that serve them more difficult, at least for the time being.

Increased Participation of Local Citizens

With increasing awareness of the link between public health and poverty, a trend called "social responsibility" also began to have a strong impact. This increased local citizens' participation in global health programs.

The term "social responsibility" encompasses *who* should be served and *how* they should be served. The "who" relates to an idea called "health equity"—access to the same quality of health care for all people. Leaders from the public health profession had long been passionate advocates for this concept, and gradually economists and businesses began to see it in pragmatic terms. As Raymond Gilmartin, the former CEO of Merck, comments: "Whether and how the world's poor gain access to the benefits of globalization will be a key factor in defining the political, business, and economic climates for companies such as Merck and Company, Inc., in coming years."[4]

The "how" relates to the voice people have in the decisions that directly affect them. The movement toward social responsibility meant those affected deserved a voice in their own health decisions, and local participation became more common in global health programs. In recognition of

"The substantial investment of the Gates Foundation, along with Rotary, totally changed the field of public health. We've gone from 'What can we do with what we have?' to 'What will it take to do what needs to be done?'"

BILL FOEGE, Senior adviser, Bill & Melinda Gates Foundation, December 18, 2005, interview

TABLE 2.1 Health spending increases in recipient countries

Country	Public health expenditure (percentage of GDP)		
	1990–1995 (average)[1]	*1995–1999 (average)*[2]	*2004*[3]
Botswana	1.9	2.5	4.0
Guatemala	0.9	2.1	2.3
Mali	1.3	2.1	3.2
Rwanda	1.9	2.0	4.3
Thailand	1.4	1.9	2.3

NOTE: This table includes the latest information available at time of publication.
1. World Bank, World Development Indicators 1997.
2. World Bank, World Development Indicators 2002.
3. UNDP, Human Development Report 2007–2008.

this increased sense of social responsibility, in 2002 the Global Fund to Fight AIDS, Tuberculosis, and Malaria (the Global Fund), an international financing institution, established country coordinating mechanisms to ensure that countries receiving funds would have representatives from civil society on the committees that made spending decisions. The World Bank also adopted a requirement for community participation.

Gradually, in response to these four trends—more resources globally, greater attention in developing countries, integration of prevention and treatment, and increased participation by local citizens—the expectations of citizens and governments in many developing countries changed. The right to have basic health needs met became an expectation, as did the right to have a voice in health services. The expectations of the developed world also changed. With greater resources available and greater participation expected, global health leaders began to have different kinds of discussions about the future. The world had taken a step toward global health equity.

FUNDAMENTAL SHIFTS IN THE ARCHITECTURE OF THE GLOBAL HEALTH SECTOR

The trends of greater resources and an increased number of players spurred changes in the architecture of the global health sector, fragmenting the traditional structure of relationships and dispersing authority. The book *International Public Health: Diseases, Programs, Systems, and Policies,* edited by the global health researchers Michael H. Merson, Robert E. Black, and Anne J. Mills, captures this transformation in depth.[5] We'll briefly summarize these changes, to provide a perspective on the challenges they pose for collaboration.

Since the mid-1900s, the structure of global health had been reasonably clear. The architecture was formalized in 1948, when the United Nations designed WHO to coordinate international health activities. With WHO as the recognized authority, global health was generally hierarchical from the 1950s through the 1980s. This architecture included the international organizations that made up the United Nations system, with relatively clear lines of authority "down" to the regional players and the developing countries being served (Figure 2.3).

This architecture was completely disrupted in the 1990s, however, with the entry of so many new players into global health and the influence of all of the other global forces that have reshaped human society in recent years. Globalization and the advent and availability of the Internet, to cite just two of these forces, created horizontal links across the globe, giving individuals and organizations unprecedented access to information and the ability to communicate with each other. Global health, like other sectors, felt these forces and responded to them.

In their chapter in *International Public Health*, the authors Ilona Kickbusch and Kent Buse capture the dramatic nature of this change. "Throughout the 1990s," they write, "the number of institutions and organizations with an interest in, and impact upon, health grew exponentially but became increasingly fragmented. The international public health scene came to comprise both global and regional agencies, including the regional development banks, the European Union (EU), and numerous national and international nongovernmental organizations (NGOs). WHO no longer played a leadership role and had become one player among many."[6]

As the influence of WHO waned, the official role of developing countries also declined. The author Gill Walt summarizes this change as follows: "States were once able to influence international health policy through their formal representation on the governing bodies or at meetings of the various organizations of the UN. However, this channel of influence no longer exists because international health policy is no longer largely decided

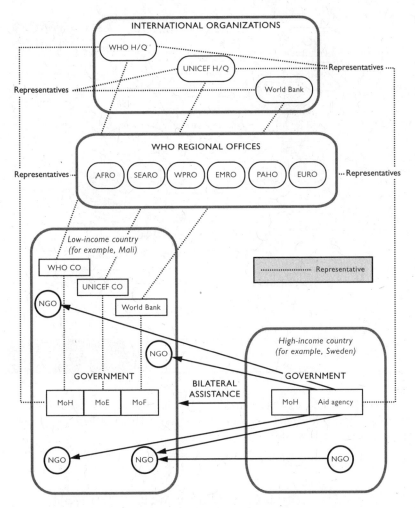

Note: AFRO (African Regional Office), CO (country office), EMRO (Eastern Mediterranean Regional Office), EURO (European Regional Office), H/Q (headquarters), MoE (Ministry of Education), MoF (Ministry of Finance), MoH (Ministry of Health), PAHO (Pan American Health Organization), SEARO (South East Asian Regional Office), and WPRO (Western Pacific Regional Office).

FIGURE 2.3 **Before the 1990s the architecture of global health had relatively clear lines of authority from UN agencies down.** *Source:* This figure is redrawn based on Merson, Black, and Mills, "Global Cooperation in International Public Health," 675.

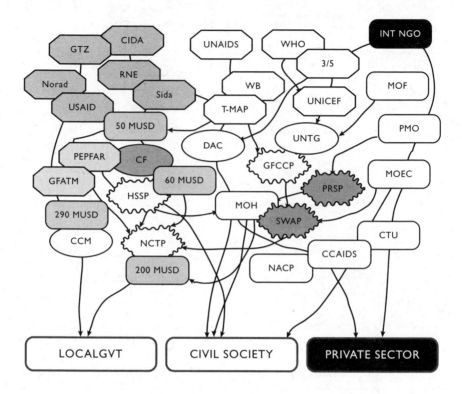

FIGURE 2.4   Multiplicity of players tackling AIDS in Tanzania, 2004. **The multi-plicity of players tackling AIDS in Tanzania in 2004 demonstrates the fragmentation that occurred in global health.**

through the UN or its specialized agency, WHO."[7] As a result, global health architecture became fragmented, with interactions and authority dispersed across UN health agencies, the World Bank, philanthropies, business organizations, bilaterals, and the country being served.

For a sector long accustomed to established roles and practices, this shift was disorienting. For example, at the October 2006 gathering Coalitions and Collaboration in Global Health: A Symposium for Global Health Leaders, Michel Sidibé, the director of country and regional support for UNAIDS, presented a visual of all the players involved in tackling AIDS in Tanzania in 2004 (Figure 2.4). The slide struck an immediate chord of recognition at the symposium. It became the symbol for the web of organizational confusion that surrounds today's efforts to address diseases/threats.[8]

Key to Fig 2.4:

International Development Agency

MUSD— MILLION US Dollars

International AIDS Programme Funders

Country Ministry
- MOH – Ministry of Health
- MOF – Ministry of Finance
- PMO – Prime Minister Office
- MOEC – Ministry of Education and Culture

National Program
- NACP – National AIDS CONTROL Program
- CCAIDS – Christian Communicators against HIV/AIDS
- CTU – Clinical Trials Unit

Global Fund or Health Sector Support
- HSS – Health Sector Support
- GFCCP – Global Fund Country Coordinated Proposal

UN Agency or Program

Development Approaches
- PRSP – Poverty Reduction Strategy Papers
- SWAP – Sector Wide Approaches

UN Oversight
- DAC – Designated AIDS Center
- CCM – Country Coordinating Mechanism
- UNTG – United Nations Theme Group

International NGO

In this new web of global health organizations, many players are not bound by the rules of the past; rather, they invent their own practices and create relationships with other organizations or governments, sending out communications and coordinating across players instead of operating hierarchically through traditional regional players and WHO. As Seth Berkley, president and CEO of International AIDS Vaccine Initative, says: "The UN is becoming more and more irrelevant when an NGO and its leader

"The structure of global health is massively complicated. . . . No one knows which meeting is most important to go to."

MICHAEL CONWAY, Director, Global Health Practice, McKinsey & Company, Inc.,
Coalitions and Collaboration in Global Health: A Symposium for Global Health Leaders,
October 19–20, 2006

can directly work with the head of state. Certainly the power dynamic is changing—in good and bad ways."[9]

Because of the increasingly fragmented relationships among global health organizations and the decline in WHO's authority, it is not only the implementation of specific programs that has been affected. It is no longer clear where decisions about overall strategy and governance should be addressed. As Walt comments, "While this pluralism of activity and partnership has raised the status of health on the policy agenda and changed the balance of power, it has also led to concerns about overlapping mandates, competition and duplication of health activities, poor coordination, and more recently about issues of governance."[10] In the absence of clear authority, policy is now being decided ad hoc by a variety of organizations. For example, since the late 1990s, the World Economic Forum has played an increasing role in trying to set the health agenda and is launching many of the new initiatives, such as the Product Development Partnership initiatives.

Bilaterals and large foundations have had the greatest impact on global health policy, by virtue of the size of their assets—particularly PEPFAR and the Gates Foundation. Both organizations are widely admired. PEPFAR is credited with bringing a systematic, results-focused approach to projects, which had been sorely missing. The Gates Foundation, with its $29 billion in assets plus a gift of $31 billion over time from the investor and philanthropist Warren Buffet, is a beacon of hope for major advances against disease. In 2008 the foundation made $2.8 billion in grant payments. While the economic downturn will undoubtedly affect future grants, the power of these organizations to control policy, by virtue of their investment decisions, creates concerns.

Global health architecture will undoubtedly evolve to another form, but until it does, those in the global health sector will have to deal with ambiguity in priority setting and policymaking.

"The world has changed dramatically since WHO was established.... The architecture's much more like a network, much more like the Internet... much more complex, and much more diverse."

IAN SMITH, Adviser to the WHO director-general, October 19, 2006, interview

TABLE 2.2 What we have, what we need

What we have	What we need
Disease-specific focus	Approach matched to current health structure
Accountability and momentum through short-term objectives	Long-term vision
Fragmentation and increased transaction costs (including time, money, the cost to coordinate versus do-it-yourself)	Harmonization for efficiency
Blurred responsibilities by each new initiative	Stronger governance stewardship and accountability
No metrics to measure the value of the coalition	Added value (demonstrated by metrics)

INCREASED IMPORTANCE AND DIFFICULTY OF COLLABORATION

Of course, our reason for exploring these issues was not to look for solutions to global health architecture, but to determine the implications for collaboration. We concluded that this new landscape—where higher expectations and fragmented architecture try to coexist—has profoundly affected collaboration. In this changed environment, collaboration is much more important but also more difficult to achieve. For example, leaders of partnerships now have the opportunity and challenge of

- seeking funding from more sources;
- involving more people and organizations;
- working harder to connect with the right ministers and staff inside countries that have undergone health sector reform;
- staying abreast of the activity of all the other teams working in a particular field, to avoid overlap;
- staying alert for where policy is being formulated in the health area of interest;
- working harder at human relationships within a partnership.

As this list indicates, it has become a much more daunting task to form, maintain, and succeed in a partnership.

When it comes to collaborations across a disease or threat, global health leaders are also experiencing greater difficulties. In a November 2005 meeting of our advisory group, Ian Smith, advisor to WHO director general, discussed the disparities between what we have and what we need to have, to be effective in global health (Table 2.2).

The landscape of global health today is more diverse than anyone could have anticipated twenty-five years ago. And with that diversity has come a shattering of the status quo that leaves both opportunity and confusion in its wake. Collaboration, never more essential than today, has also never been more challenging.

NOTES

1. PARTNERS is a coalition of Partners in Health, the CDC, WHO, and the Task Force for Child Survival and Development. The program is funded by the Bill & Melinda Gates Foundation.
2. Foege in the preface to Foege et al., *Global Health Leadership and Management,* xxi.
3. Christian Baeza et al., *Healthy Development: The World Bank Strategy for Health, Nutrition, and Population Results* (Washington, D. C.: World Bank, 2007), which sites Catherine M. Michaud of the Harvard School of Public Health, from January 2007.
4. Gilmartin as quoted in *Global Health Leadership and Management,* 9.
5. Merson, Black, and Mills, *International Public Health.*
6. Kickbusch and Buse, "Global Influences and Global Responses: International Health at the Turn of the Twenty-first Century," in Merson, Black, and Mills, *International Public Health: Diseases, Programs, Systems, and Policies,* 712.
7. Walt, as quoted in Merson, Black, and Mills, "Global Cooperation in International Public Health," in *International Public Health: Diseases, Programs, Systems, and Policies,* 690.
8. Michel Sidibé's presentation at Coalitions and Collaboration in Global Health: A Symposium for Global Health Leaders, Carter Center, Atlanta, Georgia, October 19, 2006.
9. Seth Berkley memo to authors, May 8, 2008.
10. Walt, as quoted in Merson, Black, and Mills, "Global Cooperation in International Public Health," 691.

Chapter 3 | NATURE OF THE DISEASE/THREAT

Once in a rare while, global health reaches a critical threshold in technology or strategy for controlling a disease/threat. Smallpox during the middle of the twentieth century is a good example: a vaccine had been developed in 1796, but it was the technological advances in the 1950s for delivering the vaccine—a bifurcated needle and a freeze-dried process—that made mass vaccinations practical. With these advances global health had both a product and a way to deliver it, and the modern story of smallpox eradication efforts began.

With smallpox still raging in sixty-three developing countries, scarring more than ten million and leaving a million dead every year, the idea of worldwide eradication began to stir in the halls of global health organizations. In 1958 the Soviet Union, where the disease was endemic, offered to donate 25 million initial doses of smallpox vaccine if WHO would launch a ten-year eradication plan inside its borders. When WHO published a report the following year that estimated global eradication could be achieved in four to five years through a massive effort, the World Health Assembly (WHA), the governing body of WHO, voted to launch the Soviet campaign.

A consensus was developing that eradication efforts should be expanded to other endemic countries, but efforts moved erratically. In 1961 the

WHA suggested voluntary contributions for eradication by its members, and support for a special smallpox budget began to grow. Soon, however, administrative problems at WHO sapped the momentum: the medical officer assigned to smallpox left in 1963, and his duties were assigned part-time to another staff member. In the same year a WHO-backed vaccination campaign in India failed due to the lack of vaccine donations.

Something was clearly needed to spur progress. In 1965 and 1966 three events did just that:

- The application of the jet injector helped accelerate mass immunization using the smallpox vaccine. Because measles was killing so many people in their countries, African leaders were very supportive of measles immunization programs, and the jet injector made it possible to administer both vaccines together.
- A CDC team working in Nigeria developed a containment strategy that reduced the resources required for eradication.
- The United States and Russia united to back the concept of smallpox eradication (an important demonstration of political will), spurring WHO to present a comprehensive plan for global smallpox eradication to the WHA.

The WHA responded in 1966 by adopting a goal of eradicating smallpox globally within ten years, allocating $2.4 million annually to WHO for the Intensified Smallpox Eradication Programme.

Fifteen years after technological breakthroughs had made mass vaccinations viable, worldwide interventions were taking place.

In contrast, the global experience with HIV/AIDS following technological breakthroughs has been discouraging.

Following the first CDC reports of the disease in 1981, science entered what Jim Curran, dean of the Rollins School of Public Health at Emory University, refers to as the "era of discovery": "Scientific advances were remarkably rapid—the first cases were identified and described, modes of transmission were documented, the etiologic agent was discovered, tests were developed for screening the blood supply, and AZT, the first antiviral agent for HIV, was discovered."[1] Even a vaccine seemed a near-term possibility.

In 1995 scientists announced another technology breakthrough—protease inhibitors. U.S. health officials launched a therapy of three drugs, called HAART (highly active antiretroviral therapy, made up of three different drugs known as the AIDS "cocktail"), and deaths plummeted more than 40 percent in a single year. While optimism for developing a vaccine had faded by this time, doctors in the developed world at least had a tool for managing the disease in many affected individuals.

The story was very different in the developing world. Those who tracked HIV/AIDS were alarmed by its rapid spread across the globe, destroying the lives of individuals and families and decimating economies in fragile areas. Bill Foege, senior adviser at the Gates Foundation, reflected this concern in his remarks to a gathering of health ministers in 2000: "The problem goes on, day after day. There is never a chance to regroup, as health workers die faster than they can be replaced, wrecking the social fabric . . . as grandmothers struggle to keep their grandchildren together, faced with the impossible task of providing food and clothes and school fees. Many of you have known for a long time that AIDS, in your country, is a national security issue. Now that is being recognized globally."[2]

By 2002, more than 700,000 people in the country were HIV positive and AIDS was identified as the leading cause of death worldwide among people fifteen to fifty-nine. Even though *treatment* efforts were given a significant boost by the Global Fund, by the U.S. government's PEPFAR, and by WHO's launch of the 3x5 project in 2003 (with a stretch goal of treating three million people by 2005), progress in *prevention* lagged and the virulent disease outran efforts at containment.[3] By 2006, HIV/AIDS had killed approximately 25 million people and infected an estimated 65 million worldwide, twenty-five years after the first case was reported.[4]

This is a disease that "got away" from global health leaders, turning into what Julie Gerberding, director of the CDC, calls "one of the deadliest epidemics in human history."[5]

Why did global efforts to address this disease move so slowly? The most obvious difference is that smallpox had the benefit of a vaccine and HIV/AIDS didn't. But other things also stood in the way. In terms of treatment, the high cost of drugs, the lack of an effective mass delivery method for the multiple daily doses of antiretrovirals required to treat HIV/AIDS, and the wariness of political leadership in many countries slowed efforts. In the area of prevention, progress was very, very low due to a confluence of issues, including lack of a medical infrastructure and testing facilities, the insidious nature of the infection, the poverty and stigma associated with the disease, the difficulty of changing sexual behaviors, and the failure of prevention technologies to target females as well as males.

The contrasting experiences between smallpox and HIV/AIDS highlight the fact that every disease or threat comes with its own set of circumstances that determines how quickly interventions will unfold. Our team decided to explore the circumstances specific to several diseases or threats, to find out how the nature of a disease/threat affects the challenges partnerships face. We developed a timeline of the evolution for each of the seven diseases/threats identified in Chapter 1 (see Table 1.3). These timelines tracked the emergence of the disease/threat, the technological and social advances to combat it, and the impact of efforts to slow or stop the spread. After analyzing these timelines and discussing them with practitioners who had been involved, we reached a set of conclusions about the circumstances faced by any given partnership:

- Efforts to address a disease/threat follow a common evolution, driven by the increasing ability to control the disease/threat.
- The mission a partnership chooses is largely determined by the stage of evolution to address the disease/threat when the partnership is formed.
- The challenges a partnership faces vary according to the social and political environment surrounding the disease/threat as well as the technological ability to control it.

In this chapter we'll put these conclusions in context by relating stories we heard from those involved in efforts to address smallpox, HIV/AIDS, and road-traffic injuries.

STAGES OF EVOLUTION

As we tracked efforts to address the seven diseases/threats, we began to see the same patterns that we had identified in the evolution of smallpox efforts.

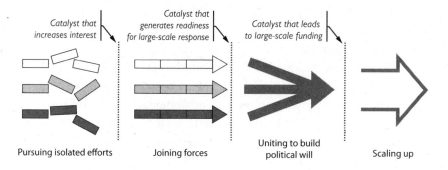

FIGURE 3.1   Evolution of efforts to address a disease/threat. **Efforts to address a disease/threat follow a common evolution, driven by the increasing ability to control the disease/threat.**

This pattern involves four stages, with some kind of catalyst (technological or social) marking the advance from one stage to the next. The primary driver is technology—the ability to control the disease/threat (Figure 3.1).

- *Pursuing isolated efforts.* The first stage begins when individuals with passion for a health issue form various core groups to address it. These groups work separately over a period of years, if not decades. (Efforts may even reach back a century or more, as with smallpox.) The focus of these early efforts is typically on generating interest, researching the issue, changing behaviors, or generating funding for those purposes. Because science has not yet developed a clear-cut treatment, solution, or cure for the disease/threat, it's harder to mobilize consistent support, so this stage typically involves a waxing and waning of enthusiasm.

- *Joining forces.* This second stage begins when some kind of catalyst— a technological breakthrough or new data on the disease/threat, for instance—creates an opportunity to control the disease/threat and sparks wider interest. As a result, advocates are able to enlist others in the cause. They solicit the support of organizations not previously involved and seek out government leaders in individual countries who welcome treatment or prevention efforts. Gradually, the number of people involved in these efforts gains critical mass.

- *Uniting to build political will.* The third stage begins when a pivotal breakthrough occurs (social or technological) that creates consensus among global health leaders that they should unite as advocates for a large-scale response. Whether the breakthrough is social or technological, a practical method of mass intervention (control) is also needed to generate widespread support. As Alan Hinman, senior public health scientist at the Task Force, told our team: "You don't raise political will until you have something you can do to address the problem."[6]

  In this stage partnerships tend to focus on building political will, for the purpose of achieving a declaration of intent for global interventions. One or more partnerships form to identify the target groups—individual politicians, UN organizations, nations, or groups of nations—and launch an effort to gain their support.

- *Scaling up.* Once the political will campaign results in a declaration of intent to address the disease/threat, it is much easier to generate funding, and in this fourth stage a rush of proposals from various partnerships ensues. Typically global health leaders have been waiting in the wings with program ideas for mass interventions, including legal changes, systems changes, or ways to take drugs and vaccines to affected populations. They soon roll out interventions.

This was the pattern of evolution that developed in all seven diseases/threats we studied in depth.

Laid out in these four stages, the evolution of efforts to address smallpox becomes easier to comprehend (Figure 3.2). The first stage began with the development of a vaccine in 1796 by Edward Jenner, leading to isolated efforts to attack the disease. The introduction of delivery technologies (the bifurcated needle and freeze-dried process) in the 1950s, combined with a 1959 WHO report raising a vision of eradication, sparked broader interest and involvement. And the development of the jet injector in 1965, allowing joint vaccinations for measles and smallpox, was the catalyst needed for generating political will. With the success of a CDC containment strategy and the adoption of an eradication goal by the WHA in 1966, the possibilities for funding opened up and interventions soon spread across all endemic areas. In 1980, WHO declared the world to be smallpox-free.

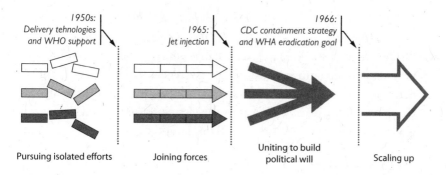

1950s:
Delivery tehnologies
and WHO support

1965:
Jet injection

1966:
CDC containment strategy
and WHA eradication goal

Pursuing isolated efforts   Joining forces   Uniting to build
political will   Scaling up

FIGURE 3.2   Evolution of global health efforts to address smallpox, 1796–1966. The evolution of efforts to address smallpox demonstrates how technological or social catalysts mark the advance from one stage to another.

For any disease/threat, partnerships form at every stage of this evolution, generating momentum and dissolving, while other partnerships pick up the baton. No single partnership is likely to play a continuous role throughout the evolution.

OPTIONS FOR A PARTNERSHIP'S MISSION

With this awareness of the evolutionary pattern in addressing a disease/threat, we began to understand more clearly how any particular partnership determines the mission it will pursue. Although any type of partnership may develop at any stage (with a mission of advocacy, research, technology exchange, policy development, or intervention), and multiple types of partnerships may be needed within one stage, we found that certain types of partnership are likelier in the first two stages and certain types in the last two stages.

The First Two Stages

Partnerships in the first two stages (when no viable mass treatment or solution is available) tend to choose advocacy missions related to research, funding, or behavioral change and health education to slow the spread of a disease or health threat.

HIV/AIDS is a good example. In the years after the first case was diagnosed in 1981 and before AZT was introduced in 1987, partnerships to address HIV/AIDS focused largely on advocacy. While one of the early donors, the Swedish International Development Cooperation Agency (SIDA), funded research and surveillance efforts, other HIV/AIDS partnerships and programs worked to raise awareness, with a goal of changing dangerous behaviors.[7] In 1985, for instance, the first International Aids Conference took place, and in 1986 the U.S. Surgeon General, C. Everett Koop, called for condom use and AIDS education.

The Last Two Stages

Once public health reaches a threshold in treatment or prevention, partnerships can gain traction in developing the political will to scale up interventions and, consequently, spur funding to address the disease/threat on a global scale. So the partnerships formed in these two stages tend to be political advocacy and intervention partnerships. Looking at two examples, HIV/AIDS and road-traffic injuries, we found that the catalyst that moved each into the last two stages was different.

HIV/AIDS: Threshold in treatment The evolution of HIV/AIDS provides a good example of a threshold in treatment that opened the possibility of building political will. As Don Hopkins, the associate executive director for health at the Carter Center, says, to generate support for disease intervention, "You need to demonstrate that you can indeed do what you are setting out to do—break transmission or reduce it drastically—and you have to have some practical tools to do that."[8] With HIV/AIDS it was the introduction in 1995 of highly active antiretroviral therapy (HAART) that proved pivotal (Figure 3.3).

With this treatment available, advocacy partnerships formed to build the political will to tackle the disease on a widespread basis, such as the Global Business Coalition. Other partnerships continued to support research in both vaccine development and treatment. The development of HAART, a truly lifesaving therapy that could theoretically be provided on a widespread basis if made cheaper, increased the impetus for partnerships to conduct interventions. When the UN adopted a declaration in 2001 expressing its intent to address HIV/AIDS, funding became available for a scale-up of programs across endemic areas. Most of the initial funding came through the Global Fund to Fight AIDS, TB, and Malaria, and in 2003 both the

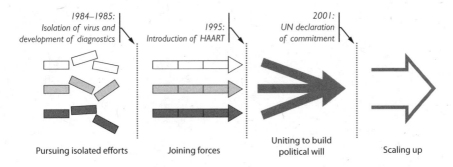

1984–1985:
Isolation of virus and
development of diagnostics

1995:
Introduction of HAART

2001:
UN declaration
of commitment

Pursuing isolated efforts   Joining forces   Uniting to build
                                                           political will   Scaling up

FIGURE 3.3   Evolution of global health efforts to address HIV/AIDS, 1981–2001. The evolution of HIV/AIDS efforts provides an example of a threshold in treatment that opened the possibility of building political will.

United States and WHO launched well-funded international interventions through PEPFAR and the 3x5 project. The G8 and the UN World Summit also adopted a goal of approaching universal access by 2010. The effort to build political will had succeeded and support for providing treatment, prevention, and care grew.

Road-traffic injuries: Threshold in data and communication   While a technology discovery prompted the shift toward building political will for scaling up HIV/AIDS treatment efforts, the catalyst for road-traffic injuries was very different. It involved a threshold in data and a new way to communicate the threat. Once this threshold occurred, partnerships had the means to develop the political will to address road safety on a larger scale (Figure 3.4).

In *developed countries* road-traffic injuries had begun to generate concern a few decades after the introduction of the automobile. In 1947 European nations formed a commission to work together in developing common signage and regulations for road travel. Rising rates of highway fatalities in the United States following the construction of a cross-country highway system in 1956 led to an outcry about road-traffic injuries, intensified by [consumer advocate] Ralph Nader's *Unsafe at Any Speed*. These concerns led to the creation in 1966 of the U.S. National Highway Traffic Safety

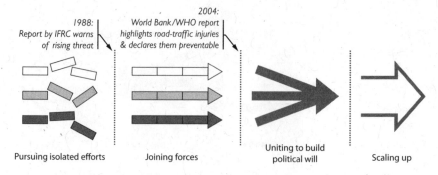

1988:
Report by IFRC warns
of rising threat

2004:
World Bank/WHO report
highlights road-traffic injuries
& declares them preventable

Pursuing isolated efforts   Joining forces   Uniting to build   Scaling up
                                                           political will

FIGURE 3.4   Evolution of global health efforts to address road-traffic injuries, 1930–
2004. With the evolution of efforts to address road-traffic injuries, it was a threshold
in data and communication that gave partnerships the means to develop political will
on a larger scale.

Administration (NHTSA), an agency focused on generating research and data and on formulating regulations.

With the increase in automobile usage, *developing countries*, too, fell victim to this problem: a 1988 report by the International Federation of Red Cross and Red Crescent Societies (IFRC) warned of the rising threat of injury and death from road crashes throughout the world. That report became a catalyst for advocates to join forces and create a stronger voice to bring attention to the problem.

As the century neared its end, WHO, the FIA Foundation for the Automobile and Society, the Global Road Safety Partnership, the Transportation Research Laboratory, and the national road safety agencies in developed countries were focusing on the issue. Road collisions were the second-leading cause of death for people between the ages of five and twenty-nine worldwide and the third-leading cause for people between thirty and fifty-five. More than a million people lost their lives every year, and another twenty to fifty million were injured.[9]

In 2004 the World Bank and WHO published a report that proved to be another catalyst. First, it called road-traffic injuries a worldwide "epidemic," a word that placed the issue in the public health arena. Such injuries, it said, were the second-leading cause of death for people five to twenty-one years of age. Second, it reported that 90 percent of the burden fell on low- and middle-income countries. And, third, it pointed out that most of those injuries could be prevented with technologies already available, such as safer roadway design, seat belts and bike helmets, and with enforcement of current speed and DUI laws. It called for a multisectoral approach for taking such technologies to developing countries.

At the same time a coalition of advocates—the Global Road Safety Steering Committee—placed the issue on the agenda of the UN General Assembly, which passed a resolution announcing that the "global road safety crisis" was a UN priority. Suddenly, the various advocates of road safety had a powerful shared language and the "bullet points" to back up their story.

Following these events, partnerships began to work more intensively at the national, regional, and global levels to build the political will to address road safety across the world. The evolution of efforts to address road-traffic injuries, HIV/AIDS, and smallpox have all followed this pattern: partnerships in the first two stages tend to choose missions related to advocacy for research, funding, or behavioral change among targeted populations; partnerships in the last two stages tend to select missions focused on political advocacy or intervention.[10]

VARIATIONS IN CHALLENGES AT EACH STAGE

With these similarities in the evolution of efforts to address a disease/threat, you might expect that partnerships would face common challenges at each stage. We found that to be true, but we also found that every disease influences how partnerships can address those challenges, depending on the social and political environment surrounding the disease/threat and the technologies available to address it.

The First Two Stages

In the earliest stages of addressing a disease/threat, the common challenges for partnerships include sociological issues because control—in the form of a vaccine or a cure—has not yet been developed, or is not yet available. During these stages people typically come together to collaborate on advocacy for research, funding, and behavioral change. The response to common challenges varies according to the nature of the particular disease or threat. The experience with HIV/AIDS provides an example (Table 3.1).

TABLE 3.1 The first two stages

Common challenges	How the nature of the disease affects responses
Determining barriers to change and behaviors needed to respond to them	HIV/AIDS: Disease carried stigma, so advocates faced social barriers to changing behaviors.
Developing an understanding of relevant social, political, and economic systems and key individuals who influence them	HIV/AIDS: Victims emerged as strongest advocates for research and funding.
Developing strategies for reaching key individuals	HIV/AIDS: The CDC and WHO identified behavioral changes needed because no drugs for prevention, treatment, or cure were available in the earliest stages.
Defining messages	HIV/AIDS: Messages were targeted at behavioral changes, for example, • use sterile needles for injections • use condoms

Jim Curran of Emory University describes the challenges HIV/AIDS presented in its early stages: "All of a sudden this epidemic began among a few gay men in California and New York. . . . When there was no good therapy and no known cause, there was fear. . . . So all of this contributed to the overwhelming stigma which still exists and is a hallmark but really took over in those days." The strongest voices that emerged as advocates for research and funding, he says, were the affected persons themselves: "Along came HIV-infected people . . . largely gay. So the role of HIV-positive persons as activists and advocates was extremely important in calling attention to the problem."[11]

Once organizations like the CDC became heavily involved, public health began to focus on identifying behavioral changes necessary to avoid infection and on considering the resources required to develop treatment. Public health leaders were driven to a behavioral focus because there was no "silver bullet"—no drug to prevent, treat, or cure the disease—in the early stages.[12]

Since the common challenges for partnerships in the first two stages of any disease/threat include sociological issues, efforts to address them

TABLE 3.2   The "political will" stage

Common challenges	How the nature of the disease affects responses
Gathering data to support a case for action (including messages)	Road-traffic injuries: A World Bank/WHO report provided needed data and framed the threat in terms of an epidemic.
Determining who and how to approach for gaining political support	HIV/AIDS: Found that strong rivalries existed within the UN system; decided to advocate for a new organization.
	Road-traffic injuries: Had to develop an understanding of decision processes at the UN General Assembly, whose endorsement was needed to generate support.
Determining key influencers and strategies for reaching them	Road-traffic injuries: Interviewed key leaders, including Kofi Annan, Stephen Lewis, Tony Blair, and Desmond Tutu, to solicit support for efforts to reduce road-traffic injuries.

can benefit from models and insights social scientists have developed. For instance, Head Start cofounder Urie Bronfenbrenner's "ecological model," which depicts various social "systems" that surround the individual and behavior, is a useful framework for analyzing these key influencers.[13] By considering the complex interactions between social systems that a partnership wants to affect, the partners can develop some useful strategies.

The "Political Will" Stage

The common challenges of the political will stage involve gathering data to support a case for action, determining what organization(s) to approach for gaining political support, and determining the key influencers and strategies for reaching them (Table 3.2). For HIV/AIDS one of the toughest hurdles at this stage was the second one: determining how to approach and gain political support from UN agencies and donors—many of whom wanted to coordinate programs and control the amount of funds the program received. Mike Merson of Yale University, who directed HIV/AIDS efforts at WHO during this time, describes how difficult and time-consuming this turned out to be: "At the outset views differed on how to approach the disease, through development or medical initiatives. There were also rivalries within the UN system. Initially, WHO was given the task but within two and a half years there was concern about the ability of WHO at the country level, etc., so the [UN Global Management Committee's] management group asked for an evaluation. In 1993, as a result of the evaluation, the countries funding it decided to establish UNAIDS. . . . And then the first few years of UNAIDS involved continued rivalries."[14] In addition to these difficulties, Merson adds, there was the mistaken belief that the pandemic was primarily confined to Western nations. As a result, "We didn't really get a global response until 1987, a full six years into the pandemic."[15]

In 2002 the Global Road Safety Steering Committee (GRS SC) faced a different kind of initial challenge in generating political will. As mentioned earlier, a turning point for road-traffic injuries occurred when the World Bank and WHO gathered and published the data to support a case for action. But to bring that case to the attention of policymakers, the GRS SC had to develop an understanding of the decision processes followed by the UN General Assembly and identify the key influencers and how to reach them. After many meetings with UN members and staff, in 2004 the GRS SC succeeded in putting road-traffic injuries on the agenda of the General Assembly.

While most partnerships are focused on advocacy in the political will stage, innovation in technology and strategy continues, and some partnerships may be piloting interventions in specific countries. For example, even while the GRS SC was advocating for increased attention to road safety among UN ambassadors, a group in Sweden was conducting two interventions that were credited with dramatic reductions in road injuries:

- *Building roundabouts.* They found that in traditional intersections with red lights some drivers will accelerate on yellow and T-bone cars coming from the other direction, creating high-speed collisions with severe injuries and death. But when traffic circles are used, causing drivers to think about what they are doing and slow down, fatalities at intersections fall by 80 percent to 90 percent.
- *Redesigning three-lane roads.* The traditional design of these roads encourages head-on collisions because drivers don't obey the dashed and straight lines of the lane markings. When four-foot

Mylar center barriers are used to separate passing cars and a "2 plus 1" passing system is instituted, fatalities drop dramatically.

After Sweden made these changes (over a thirty-year period), child deaths alone from road-traffic injuries plummeted from more than 135 a year to 1 a year. As a result, the Swedish government adopted a "vision zero" goal. Britain, New Zealand, and the Netherlands are implementing these roadway changes, and road-safety leaders now call traffic circles and center barriers "vaccines for roads" and talk about "eradicating" road-traffic deaths, a goal as powerful as the eradication of smallpox.

The "Scaling-up" Stage

At the scaling-up stage, the common challenges relate to the practicalities of taking prevention or treatment efforts to the populations of developing countries. We have identified the common challenges at each phase of this stage: (1) the research phase, (2) the policymaking phase, and (3) the program-delivery phase (Table 3.3).

The research phase. In this phase the partners are (ideally) analyzing cultural, economic, and political factors, trying to determine the best approach to implementation, to size demand for program services, to develop the needed supply of drugs and equipment, and to find funding and other resources. Although those are common challenges across partnerships, the nature of the disease/threat affects how a partnership addresses each of the challenges.

For example, one of the often mentioned efforts to combat HIV/AIDS took place in Botswana in 2001, when HIV/AIDS was a fast-growing threat, affecting almost 39 percent of adults.[16] Given the nature of the disease and the stigma it had generated in Botswana, leaders of the implementation effort decided they needed an advocacy tool. They involved several partners in developing a plan for using mass media to address the challenge.

> In Botswana HIV/AIDS was the proverbial "elephant in the room" that no one discussed. More than 300,000 people were infected, but the culture of Botswana kept the disease from being mentioned in public. While radio reports often included advice on HIV/AIDS, citizens had gotten so used to hearing and dismissing the advice that it became known as the "radio dis-

TABLE 3.3 The "scaling-up" stage

Common challenges	How the nature of the disease affects response
Determining the best approaches to implementation; sizing demand; developing the needed supply of drugs and equipment; and finding resources	HIV/AIDS: Once tests became available, it became clear that Botswana, one of Africa's richest and smallest countries, had one of the highest HIV rates in the world. A partnership with the government, Merck, and the Gates Foundation rapidly increased resources to see how it might make progress against HIV/AIDS. One of the important efforts was to use advocacy to encourage victims to seek treatment. The partnership produced a soap opera whose lead character was HIV positive. HIV/AIDS: For IAVI (focused on research), vaccine production estimates were critical, so the organization could conduct vaccine field trials without facing drug delays. It has leveraged private sector expertise to generate better production estimates for manufacturers of vaccines.
Developing an understanding of relevant social and political systems and developing the needed policies (with input from local representatives)	Child immunization: The Task Force for Child Survival needed to implement a broad immunization program quickly. To communicate with leaders of multiple counties about the needed policies, it held large conferences, attended by ministers of health and heads of agencies in targeted countries. Road-traffic injuries: Because research revealed that road safety was not a primary concern of any ministry, the Global Road Safety Steering Committee had to involve a range of organizations and ministries in policy development. HIV/AIDS: Stymied by cultural issues, leaders of such efforts are now trying to influence every sector to develop policies to address the threat.
Managing fund-raising, staffing, technical assistance, treatment, and monitoring	Smallpox: To make the surveillance and containment strategy work, public health officials devised a reward system for finding victims within a containment area.

ease." A partnership between several Botswana and U.S. organizations (including the CDC) took an innovative and highly effective approach to behavioral change.[17] Drawing on local talent, they produced a soap opera called *Makgabaneng*, in which a major character contracts HIV and goes to a clinic for treatment.

The impact was extraordinary. Audiences were mesmerized by this frank depiction of a health condition that had carried such a social stigma. Gradually, people began to talk about it among themselves and, over the course of three years, the number of people reporting to clinics rose. Follow-up research indicated that over 60 percent of the intended audience were regular listeners to *Makgabaneng*, and they were three or four times more likely to be tested for HIV than occasional listeners.[18]

This is an innovative example of a partnership that drew on research to customize its approach to a particular disease and ended up changing the cultural mind-set.

Fortunately, while partners in the scaling-up stage may include NGOs and in-country professionals (where that capability exists), they may also include multinational corporations. As Jim Austin, professor emeritus at Harvard Business School, pointed out at the Carter Center symposium in 2006, the private sector can bring more to the table than money or drugs. The Global Alliance for Vaccines and Immunization (GAVI), for example, with a mission of developing and testing potential vaccines, has a critical need to develop good production estimates for drug companies. Without good estimates it runs the risk of creating trial delays.

In a 2003 article in the *McKinsey Quarterly*, consultants Rajat K. Gupta and Lynn Taliento describe how GAVI has drawn on the expertise of the private sector: "[It] has leveraged the private sector's expertise by developing a new approach to introducing products: Accelerated Development and Introduction Plans (ADIPS). Thanks to it, the public sector can generate better forecasts for the uptake of vaccines, thereby providing a more accurate production estimate for manufacturers and ultimately, perhaps, lowering prices and avoiding the need for up-front guarantees."[19] Often, global health teams welcome corporate assistance in this phase to develop a good forecast; donate in-kind assets (such as filters for water or netting for mosquitoes); or, as Gupta and Taliento suggest, "fill gaps in the public health infrastructure by delivering health services to their employees and, sometimes, to the local community."[20]

The policymaking phase.   When research is completed and policymaking begins, the challenge is to develop an understanding of the social and political systems of targeted populations and to work with local authorities to shape the needed policies for implementation. When a vaccine is available and social barriers are low, those resources are typically ministries of health, regional and local health departments, and NGOs and community leaders who can mobilize volunteers.

The Task Force for Child Survival (1984–1990) provides a good example of working with local authorities to shape policies for implementation.

> Some eighteen months after its formation, the Task Force invited representatives from developing countries to participate in a conference that dealt with both policy and practices. The conference took place in Cartagena, Colombia, in 1985, and subsequent conferences were held in France in 1988 and Thailand in 1990. In his history of the Task Force, Newton Bowles, senior adviser to UNICEF, says, "The conferences were not intended to make decisions or formal commitments, but rather to inform, enlighten, and energize." He describes the tone and participants: "These conferences aimed at mobilizing and sustaining support for Task Force goals. Like the Task Force itself, they were ad hoc affairs, not encumbered by institutional protocol but free to range over immediate practical problems and policy challenges. Participation was arranged so as to bring together major sources of external aid (multilateral and bilateral) with a representative group of developing countries."[21]
>
> While the tone was informal, the Task Force set a standard for high-level participation. "If these conferences were to have any influence on policy and resources," says Bowles, "a high level of participation was essential; and so it was that usually Ministers of Health and Heads of Agencies attended."[22]

The approach proved to be highly effective. With strong support from targeted countries and with the resources to supplement local infrastructure, the Task Force announced achievement of the goal in 1990.

In efforts to prevent road-traffic injuries, efforts to change policies in targeted countries were very different. When the GRS SC gathered information relating to road safety in developing countries, they found that people almost universally accepted road-traffic injuries with a sense of fatalism.

The GRS SC also analyzed the social and political systems that affected road-traffic injuries within a country and found that road safety was not a primary concern of any ministry and typically fell through the cracks. A range of professionals needed to be involved in any in-country effort:

· Transportation (roadway and vehicle design)
· Law enforcement
· Urban planning
· Economic development and finance
· Education and communication
· Public health (including prevention, trauma care, and rehabilitation)

Each of these sectors had something to contribute. Transportation officials could affect policies relating to road construction and maintenance. Police could determine how strictly to enforce traffic rules and influence changes in policy. Urban planners and ministers of economic development and finance could affect traffic flow and financing of roads. And education, communication, and medical officials could help to educate the populace and other officials about the extent of the health threat posed by road-traffic injuries, plan prevention programs, and convene the various sectors. This effort continues today, and clearly the policymaking phase will be very complex.

Like road-safety leaders, those working to take HIV/AIDS treatment to the developing world gradually realized they would have to broaden their policymaking efforts. Susan Holck, director of general management at WHO, says: "At least we recognize now how big this problem is, and that we can't solve it just in the public health community. AIDS is so big and complex—it involves sex and intimate behavior—the interventions that work aren't the ones public health is good at. UNAIDS has raised the issue beyond that community."[23] Policymaking efforts are now directed at virtually every sector of affected countries.

The program-delivery phase. The third challenge common to scaling up a program lies in program delivery—the project management issues of fund-raising, staffing, technical assistance, treatment, and surveillance. Like the other challenges, this one must be met with innovative strategies at times, according to the particular disease/threat. The experience with smallpox eradication in India is a good example. The success of the surveillance and containment strategy depended on finding every case in an area where infections had occurred. To find the last remaining victims, public health officials organized search teams of public health workers and provided incentives for those who found cases.

These examples of how several partnerships dealt with the challenges of each stage of addressing a disease or threat helped us appreciate how different their responses were. When we began this research on the evolution of efforts to address diseases/threats, we knew instinctively, as do others in the global health community, that each disease or health threat comes with its own set of circumstances. We did not anticipate, however, how much these circumstances are interwoven into every stage of addressing a disease/threat. As others build on these initial ideas, we believe the evolution framework and histories of how partnerships have responded to the common challenges can become reference points for partnerships. In the following chapters, we describe how other partnerships have responded to the challenges they have faced.

NOTES

1. From the foreword in *The Encyclopedia of AIDS: A Social, Political, Cultural, and Scientific Record of the HIV Epidemic,* available online at http://www.thebody.com/content/art14017.html.
2. Foege, "Health Ministers as Good Ancestors?" 2.
3. UNAIDS, *2004 Report on the Global AIDS Epidemic,* available online at http://www.unaids.org/bangkok2004/report.html.
4. Merson, "HIV-AIDS Pandemic at Year Twenty-five," 2414.
5. Gerberding, "Main Way to Stop AIDS," A15.
6. Hinman, interview with the authors, December 7, 2004.
7. This was a partnership between the CDC, the U.S. Department of Health and Human Services, the Belgian Institute of Tropical Medicine, and Zaire's public health department.
8. Hopkins, interview with the authors, September 29, 2005.
9. *2004 WHO/World Bank, World Report on Road Traffic Injury Prevention,* 3.
10. In charting these diseases and threats, we've purposely kept the visuals simple. We recognize that reality is more complex than such charts suggest, and the events could also be interpreted differently. A case could also be made that the stages began and ended at different dates from the years we have selected. In addition, if there is a tech-

nological shift in the disease, such as the development of a drug-resistant strain, technology issues can reassert themselves, prompting a reiteration of some of the stages.

11. Curran's presentation at Coalitions and Collaboration in Global Health: A Symposium for Global Health Leaders, October 19, 2006.

12. As Curran has noted, "There are still no silver bullets, in terms of vaccine or curative therapy, and the problem of infection endures among tens of millions of people" (ibid.).

13. Bronfenbrenner's "ecological model" is available online at http:// www.des.emory .edu/mfp/302/302bron.PDF.

14. Merson's presentation at Coalitions and Collaboration in Global Health: A Symposium for Global Health Leaders, October 19, 2006.

15. Ibid.

16. World Health Organization, "Botswana: Summary Country Profile for HIV/AIDS Treatment Scale-up," June 2005, available online at http://www.who.int/3by5/ support/june2005_bwa.pdf.

17. The organizations included Botswana's Ministry of Health, the Department of Information and Broadcasting, the University of Botswana, the National AIDS Coordinating Agency, the CDC, and the Botswana/USA Projects.

18. Communication Initiative Network, February 20, 2009, update; available online at http://www.comminit.com/en/node/123510.

19. Gupta and Taliento, "How Businesses Can Combat Global Disease," 102.

20. Ibid., 103.

21. Bowles, *The Task Force for Child Survival and Development: Hope as Energy,* 6.

22. Ibid.

23. Holck's presentation at Coalitions and Collaboration in Global Health: A Symposium for Global Health Leaders, October 19–20, 2006.

In chapters 2 and 3 we've described two challenges to developing real collaboration—the diverse landscape of global health and the nature of the disease or threat. The third major area consists of the cultural and social challenges of working with a diverse group of human beings.

The formative period of the Mectizan Donation Program illustrates how easy it is for cultural issues to get in the way of close collaboration.

Africans had lived with what they called "river blindness" for generations when Merck & Co. made a key discovery in 1987. Bill Foege, senior adviser for the Bill & Melinda Gates Foundation, recalls this turning point: "This all developed because Merck in the early 1980s put out a drug for heartworm in dogs. But then a scientist got the idea this might be useful in the human disease onchocerciasis, and it turned out to be a wonder drug."[1]

Onchocerciasis had earned its nickname because the spread of the disease follows that of the black fly (host to the onchocerca parasite), which thrives in riverside areas. Infection can lead to irreversible blindness. Merck found that an annual dose of the drug ivermectin (the trade name is Mectizan) would prevent blindness. The breakthrough opened up a huge opportunity. The disease was endemic in thirty-five countries (twenty-eight of them in Africa) and had infected millions of people. In "oncho" zones 90 percent or more of the population had been infected.[2] World Bank and UN agencies were eager to partner with Merck to prevent river blindness and the economic devastation that follows in its wake.

But when they reached the stage of conducting clinical trials, a cultural clash began to appear. Merck found that its culture, which valued business effectiveness, was very different from the culture of the Special Program for Research and Training in Tropical Diseases (TDR), which had been proposed as a partner.[3] Reflecting the United Nations culture, TDR valued broad access to treatment (based on the concept of health equity).

Merck funded the first trials in 1981 in Senegal, with encouraging results. For the double-blind studies in 1983 and 1984, TDR joined Merck as a cofunder. When the results were reported in 1986, Merck was satisfied that ivermectin was safe and effective and applied to register the drug in France as a treatment for human onchocerciasis the following year.

By then the first differences in the cultures of Merck and TDR had surfaced.[4] Merck was accustomed to treatments of individuals in clinical settings while TDR and OCP (the Onchocerciasis Control Program) were focused on mass treatment using community volunteers, so they could quickly interrupt transmission of the disease. TDR cofunded (with Merck) community-based trials in 1987 and 1989. During this time Merck continued to urge TDR to take leadership in planning how the drug would be distributed. With its business orientation, Merck wanted to put constraints on distribution, requiring evidence that individual countries were capable of administering the program. That meant some countries would not have access to the drugs. Merck also wanted an intermediary to play the screening role, shielding it from such decisions. But TDR was reluctant to deprive any country of access to the drug. When TDR suggested an approach to distribution in September 1987, the mechanism they proposed did not incorporate Merck's preferences. Again, differences in the culture of the potential distribution partners had emerged, and this time it was a deal breaker.

A week later Merck moved ahead without TDR. It announced that it would form an independent committee to screen drug requests, the Mectizan Expert Committee, to be housed at the Task Force for Child Survival and Development.

Cultural differences had ended a partnership before mass interventions even began.

While differences in culture complicate partnerships everywhere, we found they are more pronounced in global health partnerships because of the broad diversity of organizations and individuals involved. These differences take three forms:

- Cultural differences across *countries* and *regions*
- Differences in the cultures of participating *organizations*
- Differences in the style, knowledge, and self-interest of *individuals*

This chapter describes the complex interplay these cultural and social differences create in partnerships. It also refers to frameworks developed by professionals in the social sciences as a reference point for understanding this complexity.

CULTURAL DIFFERENCES ACROSS COUNTRIES AND REGIONS

It's impossible today to speak of a single culture of "global health." Since the late 1980s, the sector has expanded to include for-profits, hundreds of new NGOs, public-private partnerships, and additional voices from the developing world. As a result, the traditional global health culture is slowly receding and a multicultural diversity is emerging. Three cultural forces are driving this evolution: the traditional culture of global health, the general cultural differences across countries, and regional and national differences in views about public health.

Traditional Culture of Global Health

Across the landscape of global health, the traditional culture of many health professionals remains a force that spurs valuable contributions but also includes attitudes that can be barriers to collaboration. The advisory group for this book defined "culture" as a shared feeling about what is important—values revealed through behaviors. Their frank discussions and the interviews we conducted highlight seven aspects of the traditional, medically oriented global health culture.

- *Bias toward facts and certainties.* Many global health leaders come from scientific fields, where fact and certainty are highly valued in decision making. But collaboration requires a willingness to invite opinions from partners who may not be quantitatively oriented and to make decisions under conditions of uncertainty.

- *Strong sense of turf, particularly among government agencies.* Representatives of agencies such as the CDC, WHO, the UNDP, and UNICEF feel a strong sense of organizational mission, demonstrating loyalty and dedication to that mission. As a result, they often believe their organizations hold "the answer" and feel threatened when another organization takes a lead in addressing a disease or threat. David Ross, executive director of the Public Health Informatics Institute, explained this idea further: "Anyone else on the horizon can be seen as a threat to their authority, and that can lead to an anticollaborative stance." This attitude is particularly apparent when one of these agencies controls the funding, he added. The attitude can then become, "Of course we want to collaborate . . . in good time."[5] Retaining control over turf can become more important than conquering diseases or threats.

- *Independence.* The culture of medicine places high value on independent work, and behaviors have developed accordingly. While global health leaders have increasingly voiced support for collaboration, behaviors have yet to catch up with this change in values.

- *Unwillingness to confront difficult issues.* Generally, our advisory team told us, the culture and language of public health favor diplomacy over directness. One person described it as a highly "mitigated culture," in which disagreement is not openly expressed. As a result, issues often remain unresolved and impact is lessened.

- *Bias against business.* People who choose public health as a profession tend to see themselves as doing good and business as being money-oriented. As a result, they often fail to respect what business can contribute to the management of global health.

- *Lack of accountability.* The consensus among the advisory group was that global health operates in a system that generally lacks accountability, failing to reward success or punish failure. One reason is the lack of resources: because global health has historically operated in a resource-poor environment, the needed tools, management training, and measurements have often been missing, making it difficult to hold people accountable. A second reason is that a global health coalition often involves people who are not held accountable in their own organizations for the success of the partnership, and they may lack experience and training in the practices related to accountability.

- *Partial inclusiveness.* The tendency of the global health culture is to value technical expertise over community and social expertise. As a result, recipient country representatives are often missing at critical meetings—understandable when the costs of global travel are considered but nonetheless damaging to the outcome of projects. Without the active involvement and commitment of host countries, programs go forward without the necessary ownership and may be unsustainable.

The global health leaders who discussed these issues with us also pointed out that the traditional global health culture is beginning to change as participation from geographic regions and sectors increases.

General Cultural Differences across Countries

With the growing participation of developing nations in global health partnerships, the cultural differences across countries have become a greater factor. Geert Hofstede, a professor emeritus of organizational anthropology and international management at Maastricht University in the Netherlands, has captured many of these cultural differences. Between 1967 and 1973 he analyzed large databases of employees in seventy different countries and developed four primary dimensions of national culture. He later added a fifth.[6] In his 2005 book, *Cultures and Organizations* (coauthored with Gert Jan Hofstede), he simplified the dimensions as follows:

- Equality versus inequality
- Collectivism versus individualism
- Assertiveness versus modesty
- Tolerance for ambiguity
- Deferment of gratification

"There is a dominant global health culture. All want to do good, but what you consider 'good' is colored by your culture. The issue is how to find the common ground to make the thing work."

RAY YIP, Director, China, Bill & Melinda Gates Foundation, Group discussion, May 8, 2008

These differences can create tensions in partnerships. As Anil Soni, director of pharmaceutical services for the Clinton Foundation's HIV/AIDS Initiative, told us: "It is truly hard to find common characteristics across so many actors. For example, commitment to social justice and increasing equity are widespread but not universal."[7]

Regional and National Differences in Views about Public Health

Across the world, perspectives on how to approach public health also vary substantially. Lou Rowitz, a professor of public health at the University of Illinois, points out some of the differences: "Public health has different meanings from country to country. For example, leadership is practiced differently in countries where the national health-care service is provided by the countries. In those countries there is a clinical focus, and almost all the leaders are physicians. Public health leadership does not extend to social scientists and other professions in the same way. . . . In Asia, Africa, and some European countries they put public health and clinical health together with a primary care focus. In the United States we separate the clinical focus from the public health focus. There are strengths and weaknesses in all of these systems."[8] In partnerships, as Rowitz explains, "The cultural differences must be dealt with first before you can ever deal with collaboration and discover ways to work together."

All of these cultural differences across countries and regions—the traditional culture of global health, the cultural differences across countries, and the differences in views about public health—can create serious obstacles to collaboration. We found, however, that these barriers are becoming less intense as global health leaders become more respectful of valid differences in approaches to public health in developing countries.

DIFFERENCES IN CULTURES OF ORGANIZATIONS

While regional and national cultures affect partnerships, the cultures of members' own organizations also play a big role. Earlier in this chapter we mentioned turf issues among UN agencies, but conflicting cultures among member organizations can also surface in global health, as we described with the story of Merck and TDR in the days before formation of the Mectizan Donation Program (MDP). Even though Merck found a way around that conflict by working independently of TDR, it later ran into culture conflicts with its MDP partners.

For many years Merck had enjoyed an easy relationship with its partners as they began a massive effort to rid communities of river blindness. The first partnership to launch an intervention using Mectizan had been the Onchocerciasis Control Program (OCP). They focused on West Africa, where the disease was most intense, and by 2002, with an 80 percent success rate in eliminating the disease in the area, they were able to discontinue the program.[9]

Meanwhile, a second partnership, the African Program for Onchocerciasis Control (APOC), was launched in 1995 to attack river blindness in the rest of Africa. The Gates Foundation provided a $20 million grant, and the initial partners included the MDP and several NGOs, with WHO joining soon after formation. This expansion into Central Africa brought a new challenge and, with it, a new conflict of organizational cultures that would slow efforts to prevent river blindness.

Another filarian disease, lymphatic filariasis (LF), was also prevalent in many of the areas of Central Africa, and one of the basic drugs for treating it, diethyl-carbamazine (DEC), could not be used if a patient also had onchocerciasis (river blindness) because it would cause a severe reaction. However, GlaxoSmithKline (GSK) had an albendazole drug that could be used for mass drug administration in combination with Mectizan in areas where both LF and onchocerciasis were prevalent. So the MDP partnership expanded to include GSK in those areas where LF was prevalent. This change brought two very different organizational cultures together, with predictable tension as a result. Eric Ottesen, now director of the Lymphatic Filariasis Support Center at the Rollins School of Public Health, had been working on the MDP project for ten years when the partnership reached this juncture. According to Ottesen, "Merck had a proud vision of itself as a company that based everything on research and avoided premature decisions. GSK, on the other hand, was a product of the mergers of several companies and had a more aggressive image. In Merck's view it was the wise old man facing an upstart."[10]

These cultural differences led to an instinctive distrust, which was compounded by other factors: the two companies were already in a legal battle over a hepatitis vaccine; the albendazole tablets were a hefty one gram, making shipping burdensome; and GSK had close operational relationships with WHO and several NGOs. The independence and simplicity of operations Merck had enjoyed were no longer possible.

Meanwhile WHO had ceded the steering of the program to an executive group of the Global Alliance to Eliminate Lymphatic Filariasis, but only with reluctance, and WHO continued to try to play a role. Tension mounted between the various partners. The MDP tried to handle conflicts that resulted from all of these differing organizational goals and perspectives, but the task proved to be difficult. "We should have had better conflict solving at an early stage," says Bjorn Thylefors, who directed the MDP program for many years, "but for various reasons it didn't happen."[11]

Conflicting organizational cultures had once again slowed efforts to prevent river blindness, and it would be more than a year before the project was back on track. Ultimately, their mutual commitment to helping people won out, and Merck and GSK began to see the upside in working together. Ottesen comments, "Both sides got a real kick out of feeling that they were working hand in hand with competitors, like the United States working with North Korea on a trade pact. . . . It has changed now and it is really smooth. In fact, GSK just announced they are building a new plant in India just to make free albendazole, and Merck is very impressed by that."[12] (We continue the story of onchocerciasis treatment in Chapter 6.)

Throughout our research we found that differences in organizational cultures were apparent not only across companies but across different segments of government as well as across the public and private sectors. For example, expectations can be quite different when some partners come from government agencies and others come from the private sector (Table 4.1).

To understand how strongly organizational cultures can differ, it's useful to sort them by type. No organization, of course, fits neatly into one type, but organizations do tend to have predominant bents at any given period. David Kantor, a consultant who applied systems thinking to the social sciences, classifies organizational cultures into four categories: open, closed,

"The forces that pull people apart are very strong, some of them are wired into the very DNA of organizations, and it takes far more than good intentions and kindhearted people to make collaboration work."

RUSSELL M. LINDEN, Principal, Russ Linden & Associates, *Working across Boundaries*

TABLE 4.1 Examples of expectations of agency and nonagency partners

Issue	Government agency	Nonagency partner
Who is in charge	This disease/threat falls under our authority.	Government agencies may create guidelines, but every partnership is free to create its own strategy for achieving its goal.
Roles in meetings	We can share what we know and recruit others to carry out our plans.	We can debate this point and come up with a joint solution.
Priorities	It is not politically viable to set geographic priorities.	We need to set geographic priorities to ensure the greatest impact.
Communication	In time, we'll get to it.	We will be able to communicate quickly through phone and e-mail.

random, and synchronous.[13] Each of these types is appropriate to a particular endeavor. Table 4.2 provides examples from our team discussions.

Applying these four types to global health, it's probably fair to say that most partnerships begin as random cultures, with each member feeling independent of the others. Whether a partnership should remain a random culture depends on what the group is trying to accomplish. For example, to respond quickly to a crisis, as with the December 2004 tsunami in Indonesia, a random culture can be the best solution as long as individual efforts are well coordinated. To launch a straightforward, focused implementation effort, the most efficient culture may be the closed culture, with a clear hierarchy and defined system and procedures. On longer-term, collaborative initiatives like the ones we address in this book, an open culture is useful so members can become part of an integrated team and actually problem-solve together.[14]

Even with a predominantly open culture, the partners need to retain elements of the other cultures to accomplish their goals. For project management purposes, such as establishing procedures and tracking goals, they need to draw from elements of the closed system. For creating a shared vision

TABLE 4.2 Differences in organizational cultures

Organization	Typical culture type	Description
Military organization	Closed	Under a strict chain of command, with strong supporting systems, it gets things done efficiently.
Church organization, such as the Amish or Far Eastern religious groups	Synchronous	Has values so engrained ("by the book") that various congregations do not need a lot of oversight or communication.
Software company, advertising agency, or academic institution	Random	Highly flexible, it provides freedom for individuals to explore new approaches and solutions.
Consulting firm	Open	Built around teams, it promotes negotiation and collaboration, taking advantage of diverse backgrounds of members to solve problems.

and keeping members on track in far-flung areas, they need elements of the synchronous culture. For flexibility they can benefit from elements of the independent-minded random culture. In these ways partnerships can function as a blend of cultures while retaining openness as the predominant style.

The challenge for global health partnerships lies in trying to guide a team from diverse organizational backgrounds toward a predominantly open culture. Organizational cultures, like national cultures, don't blend easily, and they can create a prickly mix on a global health project.

DIFFERENCES BETWEEN INDIVIDUALS

Of course, individuals also bring their own differences to a partnership, and such differences can pose difficulties for collaboration based on personal style, knowledge, and self-interest.

Differences in personal style may be the single biggest driver of conflict on a partnership. The Myers-Briggs Type Indicator classifies personalities into four categories of temperament, based on the theories of psychologist Carl Jung and subsequent work by California psychologists David Kiersey and Marilyn Bates: rationals, idealists, guardians, and artisans.[15] The rationals are fascinated by concepts and love the challenge of applying them in an organization. The idealists are visionary and have the gift of helping others contribute to the best of their ability. The guardians anchor an organization because they value setting a pathway and establishing standard procedures. And the artisans are inherently optimistic and may spot opportunities others miss. All of these qualities are useful in a partnership. The challenge is to lessen potential conflict through respect for all types and to develop an open culture that encourages all types to participate in solving problems.

The various degrees of knowledge among team members, both about the technical issues of a health threat and about leadership and management issues, also add to the complexity of partnership dynamics. Mark Rosenberg, one of this book's coauthors, provides a personal example of the differences in knowledge that stem from experience. In 1978 he had started a project using photographs and interviews to document experiences in a hospital and show how illness affects individuals and their families:

> I thought I knew what it was like being a patient because I had been a doctor and had taken care of patients. I would write "CXR" in an order book and it meant "take this person for a chest X-ray." Until I took the pictures, I didn't really know what it was like for the patient. I went with an elderly woman, to get her X-rays. Her breast cancer had spread to her spine, and she had to be lifted onto a steel stretcher, wheeled through the hallway,

"It's often the headquarters and those who are more distant from it that breed the greatest sense of competition because at the headquarters people are more concerned with the preservation of the organization, and I think it's the people who are at the grass roots who often need to keep reminding us that it's really not the preservation of the *organization*. It's the preservation of *life*."

HELENE GAYLE, President and CEO, CARE USA, Coalitions and Collaboration in Global Health: A Symposium for Global Health Leaders, October 19–20, 2006

bump by bump, kept in the hallway for ages while the staff had their Christmas party, lifted onto the X-ray table, then lifted back onto the stretcher to make the journey back to bed.

That process of getting the chest x-rayed was so different from the process of writing "CXR." It made me aware of the enormous gulf.[16]

If people can suffer from a lack of knowledge within their own hospitals, NGOs, and agencies, the issue is magnified when they form a partnership.

Besides differences in direct experiences, members may have disparities in knowledge due to any number of things, such as ease of access to current information, different levels of roles in their own organizations, wealth, status, gender, or attitudes toward technology and learning. All of these differences in knowledge tend to create degrees of separation. Another area of differences between individuals in a partnership lies simply in their self-interests. In any given partnership, every member arrives with a personal agenda as well as an organizational agenda. For example, that personal agenda may be to network among other partners, demonstrate leadership, or demonstrate expertise in the health threat. Until personal agendas are aligned with the larger goal of the partnership, they are likely to interfere with the group's progress.

While diversity within partnerships may produce clashes because of these differences in style, knowledge, and self-interest, it can also be of real value. These differences can enrich discussions and increase the possibilities for solving problems. When two people from different agencies or countries are in close proximity, they have a chance to glimpse each other's world, creating what has been called an "adjacent possible."[17] If a leader has the skills to increase understanding, engender respect for various cultures, and manage conflict productively, these differences between individuals can lead to the innovative discussions that characterize real collaboration.

"Relationships, or at least good relationships, don't take away from our individual identities. They add a new element, an entity that we grow to value. There's still me and you, but now there's also us. That's how collaboration works when done well."

RUSSELL M. LINDEN, Principal, Russ Linden & Associates, *Working across Boundaries*

The issues of cultural and social differences raised in this chapter are a constant source of conflict for global health partnerships. When a partnership is formed, the organizational agendas and cultures of individuals, organizations, and even nations take a seat at the table, and undercurrents of misunderstanding flow across debates. In fact, at the Carter Center symposium in 2006, Jim Austin, professor emeritus at Harvard Business School, cited culture as the number one issue on his list of initial barriers to collaboration. The challenge of responding to this human diversity has little to do with the "hard" issues of strategy, goal-setting, and measurement; it's about managing relationships on the team. As Austin points out, it may be the hardest challenge of all.

NOTES

1. Foege's comments are from an advisory group meeting, November 10–11, 2005.
2. Benton et al., *Partnership and Promise*.
3. The program was jointly sponsored by the UNDP, the World Bank, and WHO.
4. For a discussion of these differences, see Frost, Reich, and Fujisaki, "Partnership for Ivermectin," 95.
5. Ross, interview with the authors, January 29, 2005.
6. Hofstede provides a Web site for conducting analysis of various countries represented in any given group; see http://www.geert-hofstede.com/hofstede west africa.shtml.
7. Soni's comments are from an advisory group meeting, November 10–11, 2005.
8. Rowitz's comments are from an advisory group meeting, November 11, 2005.
9. Following the discontinuance of the OCP, the African Program for Onchocerciasis Control (APOC) assumed responsibility for sending Mectizan tablets to West African countries.
10. Ottesen, interview with the authors, October 14, 2008.
11. Thylefors, interview with the authors, July 20, 2006.
12. Ottesen, interview with the authors, October 14, 2008.
13. These four types are based on the Kantor System Typology and Communicational Domains. See Kantor and Lehr, *Inside the Family*.
14. Rob Lehman of the Fetzer Institution has repeatedly used the word "open" to describe such collaborations: "Collaboration, on the surface, is about bringing together resources, both financial and intellectual, to work toward a common purpose. But true collaboration has an 'inside,' a deeper more radical meaning. . . . The inner life of collaboration is about states of mind and spirit that are open—open to self-examination, open to growth, open to trust, and open to mutual action. . . . The practices of true collaboration are those practices of awareness, listening, and speaking that bring us

into openness and receptivity" (Lehman as quoted in Olson and Harris, "Defining Common Work," 6).

15. Keirsey and Bates, *Please Understand Me.*
16. Mark L. Rosenberg, *Patients: The Experience of Illness* (Philadelphia: Saunders Press, 1980).
17. This term is used in Sauffman, *Competitiveness of Nations in a Global Knowledge-based Economy,* 243.

With such complex challenges facing global health initiatives, we knew it was impossible to try to devise a simple formula for achieving real collaboration. At the same time, partnerships clearly need some kind of guidance. We asked ourselves how we could frame the lessons learned from the partnerships we were examining in a useful way.

To prepare for the meeting of our advisory group, we developed materials around a theme of "Last Mile" collaboration—stressing the importance of collaborating in a way that takes the project all the way to impact, whether that is in terms of saving lives or achieving a technological breakthrough. The individuals who assembled for that meeting were recognized leaders from WHO, UNICEF, the CDC, the World Bank, the Carter Center, the Rockefeller and Gates foundations, nonprofits, and academia. They cautioned us that the First Mile was just as critical as the Last Mile, because teams had to lay the foundations for success in that first mile.

Following that meeting, we began to explore the stages of a partnership's work, laying out the research we had accumulated on the seven partnerships mentioned in Chapter 1 along a timeline of activity (see Table 1.3). We found that the resulting Partnership Pathway helped us understand the elements that contributed to success at each stage of a partnership. Although we recognize that partnerships don't progress in the linear way a pathway might suggest, they do share common stages. By using this simple pathway design, we hope to help global health practitioners connect with their own experiences on projects and begin to consider which of the insights may be useful in their work.

The next five chapters convey the insights we've gained from this research, using this Partnership Pathway as a reference point. We start by laying out the Pathway in Chapter 5; we focus on the First Mile in Chapter 6; we examine the Journey in Chapters 7 and 8; and we turn to the Last Mile itself in Chapter 9, providing Bill Foege's perspective on this critical stage of a partnership. Chapter 10 suggests ways for donors to support collaboration.

Chapter 5 | LESSONS ALONG THE PARTNERSHIP PATHWAY

In a book about climbing the world's second-highest mountain, K2 in the Himalayas, photographer Jim Curran describes the experience of seeing the peak from base camp: "There it was, unequivocal, real, present, impassive and quite monumentally huge. A great triangle that hung like a gigantic backdrop to the silent amphitheatre of Concordia. It, too, was draped in snow and its wintery vastness looked utterly impregnable, yet with a beauty and simplicity of form and balance that gave it a certain lightness that I had not expected from the many photos I had seen taken from this spot."[1] Curran's description reminded us of the perspective of global health leaders when they set out to achieve one of global health's daunting goals. The goal is distant, the way is risky, and success is far from certain.

This chapter lays out the key elements that contribute to success in reaching that kind of goal. We identified these elements for each stage of the Partnership Pathway: the First Mile, the Journey, and the Last Mile (Figure 5.1).

To provide an overview of all the elements, we will trace the Pathway of the Partnership Against Resistant Tuberculosis: A Network for Equity and Resource Sharing (PARTNERS) effort to address multi-drug-resistant TB (MDR-TB), beginning in the late 1990s. This project, like most partnerships that involve a diverse group of stakeholders and a rapidly changing environment, had its shortfalls. Fortunately, when we interviewed indi-

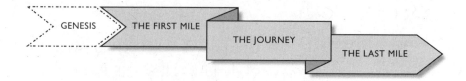

FIGURE 5.1 Partnership Pathway. **A simple diagram of a partnership's pathway to achieving its goal allows a comparison of the complex activities and interactions that occur in each stage.**

viduals who had participated, they were willing to dissect those shortfalls, to help others learn how to avoid them. "Having the experience of running this project was the most valuable experience of my life. It was an incredibly important first foray in attempting to scale up a complex health intervention," recalls Jim Yong Kim, who served as principal investigator on the project and chairs the Department of Global Health and Social Medicine at the Harvard Medical School. "It made me ready for my experience at WHO." At the same time, he recognizes, "It's not that there's nothing we could have done differently. But there wasn't a body of scientific literature on the scale-up of complex interventions that could guide us."[2] Mark Rosenberg, who joined Kim in developing the project, admits, "It takes courage to say we didn't always know what we were doing, but it's necessary if we want to draw lessons from the experience." In fact, it is often the ability of partners to adapt to external forces that allows them to succeed. Using this partnership as a reference point, we discuss each stage below, beginning with the amorphous, pre-partnership period we call the "Genesis."

THE GENESIS OF A PARTNERSHIP

The Genesis of a partnership lies in the realization by individuals that they have an opportunity to make a real difference in the world. This moment of realization typically has a catalyst, such as a report that confirms cause-effect linkages or a technology breakthrough that makes treatment more viable. As we described in Chapter 3, such catalysts occur at key points in the evolution in addressing a disease or health threat, and partnerships are often born at these points. The impetus may begin with an entrepreneurial individual who has a vision, a "social organization" of like-minded associates, or a donor organization that identifies a need it would like to address. It may even arise out of a group's desire to have its voice heard. Whatever the source, a program idea emerges, and from that seed a partnership begins to form. The Genesis of the PARTNERS project falls into the "social organization" category. Like many partnerships, it began with individuals who tapped others they had come to trust. These particular individuals, Paul Farmer and Jim Kim of Harvard Medical School, had been trying to develop a viable treatment for MDR-TB for many years. (This project took place before the identification of an even more resistant strain—XDR-TB.)

MDR-TB is resistant to the two most powerful anti-TB drugs available— isoniazid and rifampicin. Treatment is long, complex, and costly. It requires simultaneously administering as many as seven or eight expensive second-line anti-TB drugs for eighteen to twenty-four months. Partners in Health (PIH), headed by Farmer and Kim in conjunction with Socios en Salud (SES), had begun to treat a number of MDR-TB patients in Peru with individualized regimens and believed they had a successful approach. It involved using community health workers to watch patients take the drugs each day and support them as they experienced the intensive side effects. The results of this approach were highly encouraging, but funding was running out.

In 1998, Farmer and Kim approached Howard Hiatt, their former dean at the School of Public Health at Harvard about the possibilities for funding a new partnership. Hiatt suggested they talk to another former student he had mentored, Mark Rosenberg, at the Task Force. In turn, Rosenberg persuaded Bill Foege, then transitioning from the Task Force to the Bill & Melinda Gates Foundation, to join their discussions. When the four met at the Task Force, Foege encouraged them to develop a worldwide vision, with a goal of demonstrating the feasibility of their approach in resource-poor settings. That could set the stage for policy change at WHO. Excited about the broader vision, this core group began to talk about the membership needed for the project.

In 1999 the Gates Foundation agreed to fund a feasibility project in Peru to test their approach.

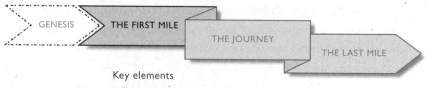

Key elements

- Choosing the right membership
- Developing a shared goal
- Selecting the appropriate structure
- Shaping a big-picture strategy
- Clarifying organizational roles

FIGURE 5.2   Partnership Pathway: The First Mile. **Like the base camp of a mountain-climbing expedition, the First Mile requires partners to consider the foundational elements and reach initial agreement about them.**

Spirits once again rose in the core team as they made their plans for the first meeting of the broader partnership. PARTNERS had entered its First Mile.

THE FIRST MILE

Because of the optimism and sense of possibility that typically characterize the beginning of a partnership, the First Mile is an opportunity that does not come around again, as many global health leaders have told us. Like the base camp of a mountain-climbing expedition, this period offers a chance to consider the foundational elements and reach initial agreement about them. For mountain climbers, this is when they acclimate themselves to the altitude, agree on their roles, and prepare for the climb. For a global health partnership, it's a chance to choose the right membership, develop a shared goal and tools to measure progress toward it, select a structure, shape a big-picture strategy, and clarify organizational roles—the foundational elements for close collaboration (Figure 5.2). (While discussions of goal and strategy might logically come before a discussion of structure, in reality, when people arrive for a first meeting, they typically want to know who will be in charge, so partnerships often prefer to resolve structure issues first.)

Below we return to the MDR-TB PARTNERS project to convey a sense of how partners can approach these foundational elements. (Chapter 6 discusses these elements in greater length.)

Choosing the Right Membership

The membership of a partnership may start with a core team of visionary people who have worked together on other issues. But that core team, like the PARTNERS core team, probably needs additional members for the project. Potential members include representatives of other stakeholder groups, including in-country champions of the affected population. (Chapter 6 discusses the considerations in choosing the right partners.)

As the core team for the PARTNERS project began to draft their grant proposal for the Gates Foundation, they discussed potential members. They decided the partnering organizations should be PIH/SES, the CDC, WHO, the Task Force for Child Survival and Development, and MINSA (the Peruvian ministry of health), which would all be needed to implement the approach on a larger scale. At this point they named the group the Partnership Against Resistant Tuberculosis: A Network for Equity and Resource Sharing (PARTNERS).

Developing a Shared Goal

The second foundational element is a clear vision and goal to inspire the members and clearly define the Last Mile of the effort. Partnerships often find it helpful to begin with a vision. David Ross, director of the Public Health Informatics Institute, makes this analogy: "As in the physical world, a partnership needs a force that 'keeps the molecules together.' If a compelling story of need and urgency is not there, you are just not going to keep it together."[3] This "compelling story" is expressed as a vision—a view of what the world can be like once the partnership completes its work.

The goal itself clarifies the purpose of the partnership, and agreement on how it will be measured makes it even clearer to partners. For example, Bill Foege recalls how public health leaders in the United States defined their goal for addressing measles in the late 1970s.

> There was much debate over how to reduce the impact of measles in the United States. Many wanted to select a target of *reduction*, such as a 90 percent reduction in cases and a 95 percent reduction in deaths. It was finally decided that the goal would be to *interrupt indigenous transmission* of measles in the United States. It was feared that a goal of reduction would not be adequate to identify the ultimate barriers.

It seemed an impossible goal and yet it catalyzed a collaboration of federal, state, and local health agencies as well as educational institutions, pediatricians, parents, and others, with the result that one barrier after another was identified and corrected. All measles cases in the United States today are due to importation; indigenous transmission has been halted.[4]

Through an exchange of ideas, global health leaders had sidestepped the seemingly powerful reduction goal and developed the non-numeric but ultimately more powerful goal of interrupting indigenous transmission.

As a core team of the PARTNERS project discussed their goal, they had the benefit of a visionary leader in Kim. He spoke of enabling victims to live productive lives in areas where MDR-TB was endemic. With Foege's encouragement, he and others on the core team broadened that vision to include all resource-poor settings, with a goal of demonstrating feasibility of their approach. As the proposed partners convened for their first meeting in early 2000, they had this vision and goal as a starting point:

> Building on the core group's ideas, they refined the primary goal, deciding it would be to demonstrate the feasibility of TB control programs that combined MDR-TB with Directly Observed Therapy Short-course (DOTS) to treat MDR-TB successfully in resource-poor settings. This, they believed, would provide a model for efforts in other high-burden countries. (A similar effort was launched in Tomsk, Russia.) They also set a secondary goal (among others) of defining and establishing the necessary infrastructure in Peru to sustain a successful program after the grant ended.

With this shared goal and a shared vision, PARTNERS had successfully established the second of the critical elements for a strong collaboration.

Selecting the Appropriate Structure

Structure discussions are also essential during the First Mile. "Structure" may mean deciding how the secretariat function will be carried out, defining the focus and composition of work groups, or any number of things that contribute to how the work will be organized. In the PARTNERS project, for example, the secretariat was initially located at the Task Force (and later moved to PIH). Working groups were also part of the discussions in the first two official meetings.

> The Gates Foundation awarded the grant in August 2000, and the partners held their first formal meeting in November—a planning meeting with breakout groups addressing clinical issues, population-based program issues (including how to arrange for laboratory services), and policy and communications issues. In early 2001 the partners met again to agree on an operating plan and structure the working groups.

In September 2001, PARTNERS refined the structure (consolidating nine working groups into six) and clarified their five-year objectives. The third element was in place.

Shaping a Big-picture Strategy

One element of structure was also part of the PARTNERS strategy. In the traditional definition of strategy as where, what, and how to achieve a goal, they knew the "where" and "what" of their strategy—they wanted to demonstrate the feasibility of using directly observed therapy to treat MDR-TB by piloting an effort in Peru. But they needed an additional element of strategy that would define the "how" of drug distribution, a major challenge.

> A critical element of the strategy they agreed on was the formation of a Green Light Committee (GLC). Made up of experts from key organizations with experience in treating MDR-TB, this committee would negotiate lower prices for second-line anti-TB drugs in exchange for deliberate oversight of their proper use.

PARTNERS, once again, had successfully shaped a key foundational element of their project.

Clarifying Organizational Roles

The last key element of the First Mile is a shared understanding and acceptance of organizational roles. With the cultural differences that characterize global health partnerships, this element is often the most difficult to build.

TABLE 5.1   Organizational roles: PARTNERS

Partner(s)	Organizational role
Centers for Disease Control (CDC)	Conducting research and setting standards
Partners in Health (PIH) and Socios en Salud (SES)	Providing treatment and collecting clinical data
Peruvian Ministry of Health (MINSA)	Developing capacity for countrywide expansion and sustainability
Task Force for Child Survival and Development	Serving as neutral convener and facilitator
World Health Organization (WHO)	Implementing Green Light Committee and setting policies

The cultures of various member organizations come into play; individual styles can create conflict; and even different language interpretations can lead to misunderstanding. When agreement on roles is not achieved in the First Mile, conflict is inevitable. When agreement is successfully navigated and members clearly understand those roles, partners can begin to build trust. In the PARTNERS project the grant proposal had spelled out the organizational roles (Table 5.1). With these roles clearly defined, the members enthusiastically launched the intervention.

The members of PARTNERS who spoke with us believe, in retrospect, they were relatively strong in addressing the elements critical to the First Mile. They had included the right members; the vision and goal had been shared; the structure of working groups had been clear and practical; the strategy had been on target in some ways (with the GLC being a key component); and roles had been clearly defined. The rest of the Pathway would prove to be more problematic, however.

THE JOURNEY

Once members of a partnership have agreed on the foundational elements, like climbers on K2 or Everest, they begin the arduous work of moving toward the goal, dealing with hazards and obstacles every step of the way.

As one global health leader remarked, the experience is one of constantly dealing with opposing forces—one force field moving you forward and another countering your every movement.

During this time, management and leadership become extremely important, as the photographer Jim Curran observed when his team ascended K2. Unfortunately, the leader of the K2 team was more interested in his functional role of climbing than in managing or leading. As Curran recalls: "Al [Rouse] was first, last and always a climber; everything else paled into insignificance.... [He] was determined to lead from the front and was pushing himself, as always, very hard, having little energy left for organizational matters."[5] As a result, an undercurrent of distrust began to emerge among the K2 team members.

The members of PARTNERS ran into a similar issue, the first sign of real difficulties ahead. Although the organizational roles had been clearly defined, members sometimes failed to fully respect those roles, and the partners never seemed to develop a cohesive energy for achieving the goal of the partnership. Alan Hinman, the representative of the Task Force during this period, reflects on the missing aspects of the partnership:

> Partners in Health and Socios en Salud were understandably concerned with taking care of the patients standing in front of them or outside their door. They didn't necessarily focus on how it would lead to a nationwide program that was exportable. CDC, meanwhile, was doing what it was asked to do, but not spontaneously asking, 'What can we be doing to achieve the goal of reaching an exportable program?' WHO thought of its role in terms of the GLC—getting money to support the GLC and the MDR-TB working group.[6]

"It wasn't that we argued bitterly or that there was any ill-feeling. Quite the contrary, as we drank the evenings away in the agreeable company of our hosts in the British Embassy Club. But there was an underlying feeling that the eleven of us were not yet making a team. Already there was too much point-scoring and criticism, rather than support and agreement. No one was trying to, it just happened, and it forced people onto the defensive."

JIM CURRAN, photographer, mountain climber, and author of K2: Triumph and Tragedy

In retrospect, it's apparent that although organizational roles were clear, some of the needed individual roles were not being filled.

The global health leaders who talked with us clarified the individual roles that are needed on any team during the Journey to their goal. In a sense all of these are leadership roles, but some of them relate more to day-to-day management, so we captured the lessons they described in two categories: bringing disciplined but flexible management and developing complementary leadership (Figure 5.3).

Disciplined but Flexible Management

Virtually every partnership we examined said they felt the need for greater management discipline. At the same time many global health leaders emphasized that management needed to be flexible to deal with the unexpected. Some of the individuals who participated in the PARTNERS project were frank about the lack of management discipline on the project. Rosenberg recalls:

> None of us foresaw how great the need would be for good management to actually implement the decisions we had made. We thought our challenge was to bring complex health interventions to *resource-poor* settings, but we realized the real challenge was delivering complex health interventions to *management-poor* settings. We didn't realize how important management was or how big the management deficit was in all of us.[7]

For example, processes for *planning* and *communicating* were conducted on the fly, and no individual partner clearly wore the hat for managing those processes.

Members of PARTNERS now see, in hindsight, that more time spent in *project planning* would have helped them understand such things as how much lead time would be required to build local lab capacity. Like any program in a developing country, they faced difficulties of infrastructure: patients were in remote areas, lab capacity was inadequate, systems for recording and reporting treatment needed improvement, and local health workers were scarce and needed training and equipment. Given these difficulties, planning was particularly important.

Hinman remembers the lack of an effective means of *communication*

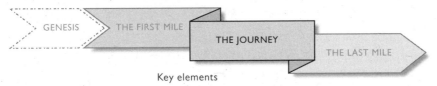

GENESIS   THE FIRST MILE

THE JOURNEY

THE LAST MILE

Key elements
- Bringing discipline and flexibility to management
- Developing complemetary leadership

FIGURE 5.3   Partnership Pathway: The Journey. **The individual roles needed on any team during the Journey fall into two categories: disciplined but flexible management and complementary leadership.**

among partners: "Mark [Rosenberg] and Jim [Kim] would talk, but sometimes they'd forget to pass it on. Some kind of explicit communication strategy would have helped, so when the challenges came up, we could have shared ideas on what we would do about them."[8] With an early focus on planning and a continued effort to keep the members engaged in solving problems and refining their plans, PARTNERS could have saved valuable time and increased their impact.

Complementary Leadership

Our research also led us to the conclusion that success depends on the ability of partners to assume complementary and essential individual leadership roles (as distinct from organizational roles). Members of PARTNERS assumed some of these leadership roles naturally. Jim Kim assumed the role of visionary/strategist, in cooperation with Socios en Salud, and Mark Rosenberg put his energies toward convening and team building. But because the partners never assumed other necessary management and leadership roles, the partnership was unable to respond effectively to some of the challenges along the Journey. For example, the nine working groups never seemed to get traction and were ultimately disbanded. That difficulty

> "There are some things you cannot take for granted; they require work and commitment. Communication is one of them."
>
> **LOUIS DE MERODE**, Consultant, Silver Creek Associates, November 12, 2005, interview

would seem minor, however, as the impact of gathering external forces became apparent.

THE LAST MILE

The term "the Last Mile" is used in many contexts in global health. It often means putting in extra effort, as in "going the last mile." Sometimes it's used to refer to the final period in the evolution of addressing a disease. For example, in eradication efforts the last mile might be interpreted as making sure the last people are vaccinated. In this book we're using "Last Mile" to refer to the final stage of a partnership, when achievement of the goal is in sight.

But what does that mean, in practical terms? For every partnership the definition of the Last Mile is different. For the PARTNERS project the Last Mile began when the partners realized they would soon have the data to demonstrate feasibility. For a project that involves a country rollout, the Last Mile may begin with the final phase of the rollout. For a research project it may mean trying to eliminate side effects for a drug that has otherwise proven to be effective. For a political advocacy project, it may begin with agreement of a key governmental group to hold a meeting focused on the subject. The keys to success in the Last Mile are adapting the approach to sustain the momentum, transferring control in a supportive way, capturing and communicating lessons learned, and actually shutting down the partnership when the goal has been achieved (Figure 5.4).

The Last Mile was a difficult period for PARTNERS. For any partnership this is the stage when centrifugal forces may be greatest—when membership tends to turn over and the remaining members often shift their focus to other efforts. The hard-won understanding and openness between members can vanish with such changes. Many people have told us about partnerships that were collaborative early in their Pathway but lost that quality before the Last Mile was completed.

In fact, turnover of the individuals serving on PARTNERS after the first two years did weaken those aspects of the partnership that had contributed to unity in the early days. Jim Kim, for example, left PIH to join WHO; Paul Zintl from PIH assumed the role of project manager; and Paul Farmer assumed the role of principal investigator. Many other members rotated out and were replaced, creating discontinuities that affected not only leadership

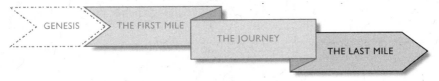

GENESIS   THE FIRST MILE

THE JOURNEY

THE LAST MILE

Key elements

• Adapting approach to sustain momentum
• Transferring control in a supportive way
• Capturing and communicating lessons learned
• Dissolving the partnership when the goal is achieved

FIGURE 5.4 Partnership Pathway: The Last Mile. **While centrifugal forces may be greatest in the Last Mile, attention to key elements helps keep partnerships on track to meet their goals.**

and management but also the culture and previous understanding within the group. The collaborative spirit that had infused the beginnings of the project diminished to the point that some of the partners felt they were only going through the motions of collaboration. These changes made the partnership less resilient in finding ways to sustain momentum and transfer control when one of their greatest difficulties became a reality—health sector reform.

On a single day in the spring of 2003, the partners learned that Peru's entire Ministry of Health was being restructured. PARTNERS had been working with individuals or entities in the ministry to develop a strategy for sustaining the effort, but now they no longer knew which individuals at the ministry would be in charge of MDR-TB. A lag in drug supplies compounded the problem. Unfortunately, the partners lacked the cohesiveness to respond with a single voice to help MINSA ensure that treatment in Peru would continue to move forward without interruptions in the drug supply.

While adapting the approach and transferring control in a supportive way were problematic for PARTNERS in Peru, given health sector reform, the partners were attentive to capturing lessons learned. Zintl recalls: "While working on the ground in Peru and Russia, we worked hard with our colleagues from both countries to coauthor papers and support their presentations at international meetings, including those sponsored by WHO and the International Union of TB and Lung Diseases. In the face of this chorus demonstrating that DOTS-Plus worked, the skeptics were no longer able to make the case that treatment for MDR-TB *didn't* work. We learned you have to work on a hundred different fronts to change policy . . . but it can be done."[9]

Zintl describes the importance of other lessons he took with him in 2005 when he went into Lesotho to treat HIV/AIDS victims once the PARTNERS project had ended:

> We went in there not knowing what we were going to find other than a horrendous epidemic—but knowing that much of what we had learned in Peru would be needed in Lesotho: training and paying community members to deliver care to impoverished patients, while also working with people at upper levels in the ministry so that ministry budgets would provide the care these patients needed. In Peru we worked with a community in Lima Norte to show that this patient care could succeed, and then we worked with the Ministry of Health so they would support that care. But it all started with the needs in the community—you can't start implementing health care without knowing what it is that patients in that community most need, if they are to be cured.[10]

The lessons had not only been communicated; they were being applied to other diseases.

Looking back on the PARTNERS project in Peru, the individuals we interviewed are enormously proud of the result, although they are well aware of the project's shortcomings. Says Kim, "We went from MDR-TB being a death sentence in developing countries to a change in perception that it was a treatable disease, even in the poorest settings." As a result of these efforts, he says, "a switch in thinking happened."[11]

> In the end PARTNERS did, in fact, demonstrate feasibility. The approach was successfully applied in Estonia, Latvia, Lima, Manila, and Tomsk, showing dramatic cure rates for a disease widely thought to be untreatable in developing countries. Initial cure rates across these programs, excluding chronically ill patients, ran between 61 percent and 80 percent. At the same time costs dropped dramatically for second-line drugs obtained through the GLC. (The GLC provided a method for monitoring drug use and making drugs available only when they're used according to specific guidelines.)
>
> In March 2005, WHO passed a resolution declaring a change in policy to integrate DOTS-Plus and MDR-TB treatment, making MDR-TB treat-

ment available to every patient, everywhere. The Global Fund to Fight AIDS, TB, and Malaria also adopted a policy requiring that all countries using Global Fund resources for treating patients with MDR-TB receive Green Light Committee approval on their projects.

The primary goal of the partnership had been met, and people across the world have been able to live longer and more rewarding lives. Since the project began, the GLC has approved more than 47,000 people for MDR-TB treatment across the world, some by PARTNERS and many others by organizations that built on the PARTNERS approach.

As the experience of PARTNERS and other partnerships have shown, collaboration is both difficult to achieve and easy to let slip away. While we found no magic bullet for developing and sustaining the open and trusting spirit of real collaboration, we did find the critical underpinnings that allow it to happen: first, getting the right people to the table, finding a shared goal and vision, and laying down the basics of structure, strategy, and roles; second, applying management discipline and playing complementary leadership roles along the way; and, finally, seeing that the partnership makes it over the goal line and hands off to the next team in a way that supports their success. (Capturing and communicating lessons learned and dissolving the partnership contribute to the success of global health in general.) As Kim explained, the "science" of scale-up did not exist when they began their work.[12] But as they and other partnerships share their lessons, the "science" of global health collaboration in partnerships becomes less of a mystery.

The following chapters cover each stage of the Partnership Pathway in greater detail and draw on the insights gleaned from successful and unsuccessful partnerships. Of course, these insights are not a formula to solve all the problems of global health, but we hope these ideas from experienced global health leaders will help partnerships improve collaboration. As these leaders told us many times, it is worth learning to collaborate well because of the impact you can have together.

NOTES

1. Curran, *K2: Triumph and Tragedy,* 40. Photographer Jim Curran is not the Jim Curran who heads the Rollins School of Public Health.
2. Kim, interview with the authors, March 10, 2004.

3. Ross, interview with the authors, January 29, 2006.
4. Foege, interview with the authors, August 16, 2004.
5. Curran, *K2: Triumph and Tragedy,* 79 and 54.
6. Hinman's comments are from a group interview with the authors on March 10, 2004.
7. Rosenberg's comments are from ibid.
8. Hinman's comments are from ibid.
9. Zintl's comments are from ibid.
10. Ibid.
11. Kim, interview with the authors, March 10, 2006.
12. Ibid.

Chapter 6 | THE FIRST MILE

Chapter 5 described the photographer Jim Curran's awe at the colossal peak of K2 rising before him when he arrived at base camp. After this initial surge of exuberance, he and his fellow climbers settled down to the more mundane tasks of a base camp—acclimating themselves, agreeing on roles, and preparing for the climb.

As we completed our research and analysis for this book, we concluded that the First Mile of a collaborative partnership involves similar tasks, and it's the experience of working together on these tasks that helps the team lay the foundation for trust and close collaboration in their journey together. As Ian Smith, adviser to the director-general of WHO, said: "The glue of a partnership is trust, yet a lot of partnerships are born out of mistrust. The challenge is to create that trust."[1]

The First Mile of the original Task Force for Child Survival (1984–1990) is a good example. Several of those we interviewed mentioned this effort as a model for collaborative partnerships, so we talked with some of the people directly involved to find out what tasks they actually worked on together in their early meetings.

We already knew about the Genesis of the Task Force, which has become part of the lore of global health.

This was a partnership born out of keenly felt need. Although WHO and UNICEF had launched an effort in 1978 to attack five childhood diseases—diphtheria, pertussis, tetanus, polio, and measles—they were not making the kind of progress they had anticipated. In the mid-1980s some forty thousand young children were still dying every day from preventable disease and malnutrition, according to UNICEF.

But new perspectives were emerging among several organizations that would lead to a new plan of attack, as Newton Bowles, a representative to the Task Force from UNICEF, points out in his history of the partnership:[2]

- Halfdan Mahler, director-general of WHO, had converted to the idea of integrated health-care delivery (primary health care), including immunizations.[3]

- Jonas Salk had challenged Robert McNamara of the World Bank to consider a global attack on infectious diseases (with immunization as one of the tools).

- Richard Lyman, president of the Rockefeller Foundation, was turning his attention to global health (and was therefore a potential supporter).

- And James Grant, head of UNICEF, was searching for an ambitious but practical goal for his organization.

They met at the Rockefeller Bellagio Conference Center on a spring day, March 13, 1984, to decide how to reenergize efforts to improve child health.[4] The heads of major bilaterals joined them, along with health officials from Colombia and Senegal. Bill Foege, the former director of the CDC, facilitated the meeting.

The mood turned somber as the conference proceeded. Ralph (Rafe) Henderson, director of WHO's Expanded Program on Immunization, reported that in 1983 (five years after the immunization project had been launched) only 30 percent of infants in the developing world were being fully immunized for DPT, 24 percent for polio, and 14 percent for measles. Those attending the conference were discouraged. They wanted to push forward with the earlier goal, 80 percent immunization of the world's children by 1990, but how could they make that happen in the next six years at the rate they were going?

A recommendation from Mahler and Grant gave them the answer: they

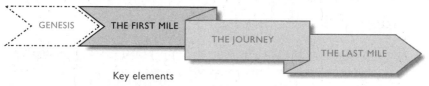

Key elements

- Choosing the right membership
- Developing a shared goal
- Selecting the appropriate structure
- Shaping a big-picture strategy
- Clarifying organizational roles

FIGURE 6.1   Partnership Pathway: The First Mile. **As partners debate the key elements that lay the foundation for their work, they have the opportunity to evolve from politeness to open expression of differences to trust.**

would form a high-level Task Force for Child Survival to bring new life to their efforts. Bill Foege would become executive director, heading the secretariat from an office at the Carter Center. A core group of institutions— UNICEF, the Rockefeller Foundation, WHO, the UNDP, and the World Bank—would become member organizations, with their representatives on the steering committee. "The stakeholders entered the villa skeptical and mistrustful and left four days later with a positive attitude toward the possibility of collaboration," recalls Alan Hinman, then director of the Immunization Division at the CDC.[5]

From that hopeful beginning, the Task Force for Child Survival continued to gain impetus.

Using the Task Force as a reference point, this chapter describes how partnerships can lay the foundation for close collaboration in the First Mile through thoughtful discussions of the key elements mentioned in Chapter 5 (Figure 6.1). Ideally, discussions of these elements take place over several two- or three-day sessions. As Hinman (now a senior public health scientist with the Public Health Informatics Institute) explained, "Dedicated meetings over several days allow members to grow as a group and generate consensus." It is during these debates that members evolve from politeness to open differences of opinion and, if they are participating in a collaborative spirit, to emerging trust and high performance.[6]

CHOOSING THE RIGHT MEMBERSHIP

The first discussion is often about membership. Years ago, the membership of a global health partnership was likely to consist entirely of a core team of people who had worked together during earlier stages of tackling the disease/threat or in addressing other issues. Today the World Bank points to an increasing tendency for partnerships to follow the "stakeholder model" (including developing countries, NGOs, and the private sector) as opposed to the "shareholder model" (with members being limited to sponsors and funders).[7] This expansion of membership presents a greater challenge to the cohesiveness of a partnership. To guide a core team in developing the kind of membership that can become an integrated team and achieve high performance, we found three considerations are important: (1) defining stakeholder groups critical to the effort and determining whether their representatives should participate as members or in other forums, (2) looking for individuals with the leadership skills needed to accomplish the tasks of the partnership, and (3) limiting membership to a size that allows for interaction, decision making, and trust building.

Defining Critical Stakeholder Groups

As our advisory group pointed out, the stakeholders who need to be involved depend on the type of partnership (Table 6.1). The two types of partnership that require the broadest stakeholder involvement are general advocacy efforts and interventions.

General advocacy partnerships These partnerships need to gather input from all segments of society because the input is essential in planning their communications efforts and in generating broad support. For example, John Hardman, president and CEO of the Carter Center, pointed out that the mental health partnership at the Carter Center includes repre-

> "A common problem of many failed programs is they haven't resolved key components in the first mile. They have unrealistic expectations, no mutually agreed goals, no clear strategy, and too little trust."
>
> IAN SMITH, Adviser to the WHO director-general, December 28, 2005, interview

TABLE 6.1   Examples of stakeholders by type of partnership

Purpose of partnership	Typical stakeholder groups
General advocacy and education	All segments of society, to provide input on how to raise awareness and change risky behaviors
Research and development	Organizations with technical or scientific expertise Communities at risk
Advocacy to generate political will	Government officials and those who influence them
Intervention	Representatives from the recipient country's government, civil society, and private sector, to plan and execute the intervention Organizations providing goods and supplies, such as pharmaceuticals and NGOs

sentatives of fifty to sixty groups, because the issue is so diverse in terms of people affected, the range of illnesses, and the settings in which it can be addressed.[8] (Clearly, a partnership of that size will not be able to build close collaboration across the entire membership, but will need to rely, instead, on a core group to develop cohesiveness and trust.)

Hardman's emphasis on including affected populations is a theme we heard frequently from global health leaders, particularly in projects in developing countries. As Ray Yip of the Gates Foundation points out: "The bride is often not at the wedding."[9] Don Berwick, CEO of the Institute for Healthcare Improvement, says: "In the end we are guests. We're in *their* houses, and I think you've got to start with the questions 'What do *you* want? What do *you* need?' The goals must be the goals of the nations in the South we are trying to help."[10]

Partnerships conducting interventions   These partnerships need to include in-country groups of stakeholders as well as organizations providing goods and services, such as pharmaceutical companies and NGOs. Awa Marie Coll-Seck, the executive director of the Roll Back Malaria Partnership (RBM), says this partnership suffered from the lack of in-country perspective when it tried to promote a change in malaria treatment in African countries in the early 2000s. She explains:

Global health leaders had known about the growing problem of chloroquine resistance for several years, and WHO had issued recommendations for a new treatment approach for malaria. But for three years, ministers of health in affected countries failed to act on the recommendations. . . . The minister of health in Sudan told the RBM board: "It is good to give us recommendations, but our problems are multiple. This is a problem of health worker training, procurement, and distribution. If you are not taking them into account, we will never implement this change in policy." He went on to challenge the board by asking if we were really trying to help countries or just trying to impose our recommendations on them.[11]

The RBM board responded by focusing on the practical implementation issues the minister had raised, and the partnership began to make headway with the new policy.

The lesson Coll-Seck drew from the experience is that in-country representatives of the area *must* be part of the decision process so their problems can be taken into account. "Simply involving the 'right' partners won't lead to success," she says. "In fact you need more than the classic partners at the table."[12]

Once a partnership has defined key stakeholder groups, it must consider which groups are needed as members and which should participate in such forums as conferences, advisory groups, or community gatherings. Three criteria for determining organizational membership are the knowledge and resources the organization can provide, its influence in the community or government, and the importance of buy-in from that stakeholder group.[13]

Looking for Individuals with Needed Skills

The core team can also improve the partnership's chances for close collaboration by considering, whenever possible, not just organizations that should be represented but the individuals from those organizations who can provide the following qualities and skills:

1. *Alignment of personal agendas with the goals of the partnership.* Our advisory group emphasized the importance of thinking through personal agendas. "In a partnership, members are intrinsically challenged to set aside their egos and concern for their own identities and turf," says Pascal Villeneuve, chief of the health section

in UNICEF's Programme Division. "That's why it's important to understand the motivation that drives each member, including organizational and personal goals."[14]

2. *Experience and technical or functional skills.* Diversity in skills and perspectives (technical, problem-solving, and interpersonal) helps the team cover all the leadership roles needed to achieve close collaboration.

3. *Positive attitude and team orientation.* It's also important to have members who are team-oriented and optimistic enough to believe they can change things. As Bill Foege says, "Optimism is infectious and spreads from the top down. There is a place for negativism and cynicism, but contract out for it. It can ruin your day."[15]

4. *Influence and authority.* Clearly, it's also important that individual members have influence and authority within their own organizations so they can tap needed resources.

5. *Emotional intelligence (EQ).* Frequently, the people we interviewed mentioned emotional intelligence as a critical skill. As Nana Twum-Danso, associate director of the Mectizan Donation Program, told us, "Oftentimes, coalitions bring together technically strong people who may not have the emotional intelligence needed."[16]

Although these are the skills and qualities that best support close collaboration, a full slate is not essential at the start. Jon Katzenbach and Douglas Smith, authors of *The Wisdom of Teams*, say: "In our research, we did not meet a single team that had all the needed skills at the outset.... As long as the skill *potential* exists, the dynamics of a team can cause that skill to develop."[17]

"In developing countries, because of their situation they are more willing to say, 'Yes, come in, we want your help,' but they may be passive. Without the active involvement and commitment of the host country, the effort is likely to fail."

SETH BERKLEY, President, International AIDS Vaccine Initative (IAVI), October 11, 2005, advisory group meeting

Limiting Membership to a Manageable Size

A third consideration is the size of the partnership. A tension exists between looking for the right stakeholders and limiting the number of members. For partnerships that want to form an integrated team, membership needs to be relatively small to increase the likelihood that every person will participate in discussions and decisions. The magic number seems to be somewhere between five and thirty, preferably closer to the small end of that spectrum. Katzenbach and Smith point out that "10 people are far more likely than fifty to successfully work through their individual, functional, and hierarchical differences toward a common plan and hold themselves jointly accountable for the results."[18]

Unfortunately, many partnerships go well beyond the ideal size. As Seth Berkley, president of the International AIDS Vaccine Initative (IAVI), says, "The UN way is politically correct, with the UN family sitting at the table. For example, you could go to a global meeting with a hundred people. This level of political correctness can paralyze work in international health."[19]

With these considerations as a reference point, we looked back at Bowles's history of the partnership and the minutes of meetings to see how the original Task Force handled membership in its First Mile.

Official membership was limited to representatives of the five organizations that made up the steering group plus the secretariat; this core group was convinced they needed to maintain a small decision-making body.[20] In Bill Foege's opinion, "If you try to cast the net too far you get to an

---

"Common sense tells us that it is a mistake to ignore skills when selecting a team. A team cannot get started without some minimum complement of skills, especially technical and functional ones. And no team can achieve its purpose without developing all the skill levels required. Still, it is surprising how many people assemble teams primarily on the basis of personal compatibility or formal position in the organization."

JON R. KATZENBACH, Senior partner, Katzenbach Partners

DOUGLAS K. SMITH, Executive director, Punch Sulzberger Leadership Program, Journalism School, Columbia University, *Wisdom of Teams*

unwieldy size. With the Task Force, six voting members [including the secretariat] made it possible for people to be heard and to have discussion. With thirty people you can't hash things out and come to agreement."[21]

But the Task Force was concerned about the lack of representation by other key stakeholders, a topic that came up in its second meeting (July 1984). Instead of increasing membership, they decided to internationalize and expand their base through conferences. Bowles describes the broadening of stakeholders over time: "The thirty-four participants in the 1984 conference [in Cartagena] came mostly from UN and bilateral aid agencies with only three from developing countries. Ninety came to Talloires in 1988, including twelve from ten developing countries. Over a hundred attended the Bangkok Conference in 1990, with forty-six persons from ten developing countries. . . . The Conferences were not intended to make decisions or formal commitments but rather to inform, enlighten, and engage."[22]

He quotes Kenneth Warren of the Rockefeller Foundation, who opened the Cartagena Conference by telling participants, "The Task Force is your baby! It is rising up as a symbol of your will."[23] Not only did the conferences involve country representatives, the later conferences also included pharmaceutical companies, who would be instrumental in reducing the cost of vaccines.

With the conferences as a way to include other stakeholders, the partners were able to keep the partnership itself small.

We recognize that forces are typically at work to constrain an objective approach to membership. Every new project starts with a great sense of urgency because people are suffering every hour from the disease or health threat, and political pressures also come into play. One of the lessons of our research, however, is that the First Mile is the primary opportunity for a partnership to involve the right people—the ones who will not simply attend meetings and occupy chairs, but who will personally help the partnership reach its goal.

DEVELOPING A SHARED GOAL

A second key task of the First Mile is developing a goal that is really shared across the partnership. The reports we read and the people we interviewed indicated that although the goal may be described in the grant proposal, it never actually becomes a shared goal in many partnerships. According to a 2004 UK Department for International Development (DFID) report, "Shared goals and objectives, together with clearly defined roles and responsibilities, are pre-requisites of effective partnership. However, this principle is routinely violated in [global health partnerships]."[24]

Several polarities may exist in the minds of partners that lead to different interpretations of the partnership's goal, such as cure versus prevention, market orientation versus human-rights orientation, or civil society involvement versus representation by government officials only. The risk to a partnership occurs when such differences in views about a goal are never surfaced. Without a shared goal, partners haven't really defined their Last Mile, and their chance of completing it is severely compromised.

The global health leaders we interviewed mentioned two activities that can help partners develop a goal they feel passionate about and understand as a team. The first is to discuss the vision or mission behind the effort, and the second is to refine the language of the goal together.

Vision

It is the vision, more than any other factor, that transforms partnerships from purely rational entities into inspired teams. When one of the partners "paints a dream," the members begin to have a collective vision, and that brings a shared meaning to the goal. As Lucy Davidson, the director of the suicide prevention program of the Task Force, says: "If you can help people visualize the potential, you can help to make it real in their minds. This is very powerful."[25]

The partnership we have been examining in this chapter, the original Task Force for Child Survival, is an excellent example of the power of an inspiring vision. In Bowles's history of the partnership, he cites a powerful vision statement by Kenneth Warren of the Rockefeller Foundation: "The children of this world will no longer be killed, blinded, mentally incapacitated and crippled by measles, tetanus, diphtheria, whooping cough and poliomyelitis."[26]

Language or Topics Relating to the Goal

Another way for partners to develop a shared understanding of a goal is to discuss its language. Because language differences can easily create misunderstandings, some partnerships debate the meaning of each word. Others arrive at a shared meaning by discussing such topics as affected populations, timeframe, milestones, and measurements of success. For example, the Task Force identified the National Immunization Days as milestones. A discussion of the projected outcome of 80 percent immunization also helped clarify the meaning of their goal. Through these discussions they began to develop an understanding of the goal that was shared.[27]

The goal of immunizing 80 percent of the world's children by 1990 gave the Task Force focus. Within months of their launch, the partnership had held three National Immunization Days in Colombia, reaching approximately 820,000 of 1,000,000 children. Jim Grant, the executive director of UNICEF at the time, said: "The lesson is the importance of quantified, time-limited, doable but ambitious targets."[28]

Whether the discussions are about the vision or the language and topics relating to the goal, it is the respectful exchange of ideas that helps a partnership ensure that everyone understands and supports the goal's meaning.[29]

SELECTING AN APPROPRIATE STRUCTURE

Once the partners gather for the first meeting, one of the issues that hovers around early discussions is how to structure the partnership. While it might seem natural to develop a strategy before turning to discussions about structure, partners inevitably feel some tension about their relative power in the partnership (and the power of their organizations) and often find it difficult to make progress until the issue of structure has been resolved.

When partnerships fail to clarify how they will be structured, these tensions can simmer throughout their work together. For that reason an early discussion of structure, based on potential models, helps a partnership move forward. In researching the common structures used in global health partnerships, we found that the appropriate choice of both the overall governance model and the supporting structures depends on the group and the goal before them.

Overall Governance Models

In a 2002 article published by the Gates Foundation, a team from McKinsey & Company cited five structural models common to global health alliances.[30] Two of these models—known as "lead partner" and "secretariat"—

TABLE 6.2 Governance models relevant to close collaboration

Model	Description	When appropriate	Example
Informal organization	Everyone at the table makes decisions.	Small number of partners (four to six) working informally Individual partners have distinct skills, for example, facilitation, political lobbying.	Global Road Safety Steering Committee (2002–2004)
Lead partner	Member from one agency serves as convener and/or administrator.	Small number of partners If the lead partner serves as the convener, that partner is able to lead without dominating discussions and work at least half-time. If the lead partner serves as the administrator, that organization is able to provide a funding path.	PARTNERS (2000–2006)
Secretariat	Head of secretariat serves as the convener and (with staff) as the administrator.	Funding provides for secretariat staff. Core partners carry major leadership responsibilities in their own organizations. The timeframe is short. Members come from the political sector.	Task Force for Child Survival (1984–1990) Global Polio Eradication Initiative
Hub and spoke with secretariat	Small groups take independent action, with the central hub acting as secretariat to integrate knowledge and coordinate action.	A small group of partners Working groups with strong leadership, initiative, and goals	Global Polio Eradication Initiative (1988 cont.): a virtual secretariat representing the partnering organizations

are relevant to the close collaboration described throughout this book. In Table 6.2 we've broadened their definition of "lead partner" to accommodate some of the partnerships we've examined, and we've added two other models that we encountered in our research: these are characterized as "informal leadership" and "hub and spoke."[31] These models depict a growing degree of organizational structure in a partnership. As the Task Force for Child Survival and the Global Polio Eradication examples illustrate, some of these models overlap.

A discussion around such models during the First Mile helps partners clarify how they will work together. In the case of the Task Force for Child Survival, the five partnering organizations funded the costs of the secretariat offices, staff, publications, and travel. By having a secretariat that was not hosted by a member organization, partners were able to keep the partnership independent. "Through the magic of neutral turf," recalls Alan Hinman, "they checked their egos at the door and were able to work through issues."[32] Bowles described the way the partnership functioned:

> The Task Force was an ad hoc arrangement. It was not caught in the sterile formalities of much inter-agency machinery. In effect, it made itself up as it went along. Under the wise guidance of its Executive Director, Dr. Bill Foege, and his steady helmsman, William Watson, from the start there was good order, continuity, and predictability in its work. The work-a-day arrangements that facilitate substantive discussion were exemplary. A formal agenda based on concerns of the whole group or of individual members was established in advance. Background papers on important topics were also circulated. A summary report of discussions and decisions was prepared after each meeting and sent to participants. Within this structured setting, meetings were informal. This was a small congenial group, [sitting] face to face around the table. It was understood that free discussion of sensitive issues would be treated confidentially, and it usually was.[33]

Although Bowles describes the arrangement as "ad hoc," elements of structure were clearly in place. Foege comments further on how the Task Force handled discussions of structure: "Organizational structure is key, but the formal effort spent defining it needs to be minimal or you harm the social capital."[34] These models, gleaned from interviews with global health leaders and from literature about global health partnerships, provide good reference points for an early First Mile discussion about governance. Some partnerships also establish a decision-making protocol.[35]

Supporting Structures

In addition to an overall governance model, a partnership often needs supporting structures that facilitate input, decision making, and/or implementation. We found a number of these structures among the partnerships we studied (Table 6.3). A board or steering committee is particularly relevant to global health because partnerships often include so many stakeholders that decision making becomes unwieldy. Senior champions are also common, as a way to tap resources and funding at member institutions. The Task Force for Child Survival used both of these supporting structures: each of the five founding institutions appointed a representative to the board, and the board became the decision-making body for the partnership; the heads of the five agencies also played the role of senior champions, especially Jim Grant at UNICEF. Hinman recalls: "He would call the heads of the other sponsoring agencies and twist their arms."[36]

Subteams, such as technical committees, working groups, and country coordinating bodies, are useful for tackling specific goals or issues. They're especially important to partnerships too large to develop close collaboration. With the support of the partnership such subteams can become the de facto collaborations. As Katzenbach and Smith say, "Extending the benefits of a team to a large group is better accomplished by challenging subsets of the group to tackle significant performance goals and then helping those subgroups to become real teams." They add, "One real team in the midst of a large group will influence overall group performance more effectively than any number of mission or teamwork statements."[37] Of course, supporting structures are not needed for every project. But large partnerships may find these examples a useful reference point for discussing possibilities.

SHAPING A BIG-PICTURE STRATEGY

Another important task in the First Mile phase is deciding on a strategy. As several global health leaders have pointed out, a strategy process can become paralysis by analysis, and that is clearly not the way a partnership should

TABLE 6.3 Examples of supporting structures

Structure	Role	Example
Board or steering committee	Makes policy decisions (with input from other partners or advisers and, as relevant, from technical committees)	Task Force for Child Survival (1984–1990)
Senior champions	Secure resources and commitments; look for opportunities	Jim Grant's role in the Task Force for Child Survival effort
		Rotary representatives in the Global Polio Eradication Initiative effort
		David Ward in the Global Road Safety Steering Committee
Technical committees	Recommend scientific decisions to board	Green Light Committee (for the Stop TB Partnership)
Working groups	Explore issues and recommend policies	Stop TB Partnership
		UN Road Safety Collaboration
Stakeholder forums	Provide insights into local attitudes and practices	Task Force for Child Survival (1984–1990)
Country coordinating bodies	Provide a coordination mechanism at the country level	GAVI's Inter-Agency Coordinating Committees
		GFATM's Country Coordinating Mechanism

begin its work. In the First Mile a partnership needs directional agreement—a simple statement of *where* the partnership will focus its efforts (for example, geography and/or target population), *what* they will do, and *how* they expect to achieve their goal(s). Discussions of these topics helps the partnership calibrate its expectations for resources, roles, and targets.

Again, looking at the original Task Force for Child Survival provides some useful insight. Strategy was an immediate topic of discussion at the Task Force because earlier efforts to achieve the same goal had stalled.

> [In his history of the Task Force] Bowles comments that "although [the leaders at] Bellagio had handed the Task Force a broad mandate, everyone knew that the first challenge was strategic: where to attack and how to win the next battle in the long war for child health."[38]
>
> In the first meeting of the Task Force, the partners clarified the "where": they would focus in the first year on the areas where the partnering organizations had already been working: Colombia, India, and Senegal. Based on the experiences in those countries, they would expand their efforts.
>
> The "what" was a given for the Task Force: they would focus on vaccinating children against the five diseases already identified by the partnering organizations.
>
> The "how" included an improved approach to operations and vaccines. Bowles reports: "Task Force attention was directed to applied research in two directions: (1) operations, including management, motivation, surveillance, and logistics; (2) vaccines, their efficacy, new vaccinology, greater simplicity of immunization, availability, costs."[39]

This strategy showed good results. "By the time of the Cartagena Conference, eighteen months after Bellagio," writes Bowles, "global coverage was climbing, and Dr. Henderson [director of WHO's Expanded Program on Immunization] was able to predict that by 1990, coverage in developing countries would reach 60 percent to 70 percent."[40]

Like the Task Force for Child Survival, every project has limited resources, so a partnership's strategy needs to make clear choices about the where, what, and how aspects of its focus. Table 6.4 highlights strategies from two other global health partnerships, as well as from the Task Force.

Once a partnership has made clear choices about the where, what, and

TABLE 6.4 Examples of strategies

Partnership	Strategy
The 1973–1975 partnership to eliminate smallpox in India between WHO, the CDC, and India's ministry of health	**Where:** India's two most impoverished and populous states, Uttar Pradesh and Bihar **What:** Using smallpox vaccinations to prevent spread and eliminate the disease **How:** Surveillance to detect outbreaks, containment of each outbreak within a "ring," and vaccinations within the ring to contain the spread
The 2003–2005 Roll Back Malaria Partnership between Red Cross, national federations, various NGOs, Exxon Mobil, WHO, and UNICEF	**Where:** Population of Togo **What:** Distribution of insecticide-treated nets **How:** Integrating effort with the existing measles immunization program
The Task Force for Child Survival (1984–1990) partnership between UNICEF, the Rockefeller Foundation, WHO, the UNDP, and the World Bank	**Where:** (in first year) Colombia, India, and Senegal **What:** Immunization against six childhood diseases **How:** Improving vaccine delivery through closer collaboration and joint planning

how of its strategy, it can agree on key actions and timing. These actions provide the basis for developing an operating plan, including funding. Foege recalls the impact of the Task Force's plan:

> Once the outside world saw that we had a global plan for immunization, it made it possible to invest in something. [Robert] McNamara [of the World Bank] had talked about upping the ante to 100 million new dollars and everyone thought he was unrealistic. Two years later, no one would have settled for that. Italy alone gave more than $100 million. . . . Once established, the Task Force changed what people were willing to do based on the plan.[41]

Although the Task Force for Child Survival inherited its goal from previous efforts by the partners, the development of a new strategy in its First Mile had been pivotal.

When members create clear strategies in the First Mile, they not only open up funding possibilities; they also generate more willingness among members to collaborate.[42] As Dave Ross of the Public Health Informatics Institute told us, "When there is a loose or poor identification of the problem, the problem isn't viewed by many people to be a problem. But as belief in the problem grows and real solutions become clear, so does the willingness for people to collaborate."[43]

CLARIFYING ORGANIZATIONAL ROLES

The fifth element partners should explicitly address in the First Mile is the roles member organizations will play. Many of the global health leaders interviewed referred to the "mitigated" culture of global health (as described in Chapter 4). They explained this as a sense that everyone in global health is committed to good work, so it can seem rude to talk about responsibilities. So partners tend to be polite and avoid bringing up such topics. But when organizational roles are not clarified, individual partners make their own assumptions about what level of staff, facilitators, or funding member organizations are willing to provide. These assumptions can become land mines as the project continues.

To prevent that kind of problem, the convener needs to make sure a discussion of organizational roles takes place. For example, in the Roll Back Malaria project the clear understanding of roles by the partnering agencies was a major factor in the project's success in Tanzania.

TABLE 6.5   Organizational roles: Roll Back Malaria

Partner	Organizational role
Exxon Mobil	Contribute raw material
Sumitomo	Provide technology to Tanzania
UNICEF	Handle distribution
WHO	Provide policy advice

TABLE 6.6 Organizational roles: Global Polio Eradication Initiative

Partner	Organizational role
The CDC	Manage surveillance network
Rotary	Raise funds in developed countries
	Build government relationships in recipient countries
	Mobilize volunteers in developing countries
UNICEF	Facilitate vaccination-day efforts
	Communicate with stakeholders
WHO	Set norms and standards (through an advisory group)

The objective was to transfer the technology of long-lasting insecticide-treated nets from Japan to Tanzania. Working under the umbrella of RBM, the partners had no official Memorandum of Understanding, and they met primarily through teleconferences. But, according to Awa Marie Coll-Seck, executive director of the program, "everybody was clear about what they had to do."[44] Table 6.5 lays out their respective organizational roles. Within two years the technology had been successfully transferred, and manufacturing began in Tanzania.

"This project was successful," Coll-Seck adds, "because all of the partners were very clear about their roles and what they would give to the collaboration, and they respected each other."[45]

The partners in the Global Polio Eradication Initiative had similar comments. As David Heymann, who is currently in charge of polio eradication at WHO, says, "Each partner has carved out its comparative advantage and sticks to that."[46] These organizational roles are shown in Table 6.6. Like Coll-Seck, Heymann attributes much of the success of the partnership to this clarity of roles.

In looking at the Task Force for Child Survival, we found the members preferred working together informally, drawing on technical and financial

TABLE 6.7 Organizational roles: Task Force for Child Survival (1984–1990)

Partner	Organizational role
The Rockefeller Foundation	Technical advice
The UNDP	Formal endorsement of decisions
UNICEF	Administrative lead partner
	Field implementer
	Funder for vaccines
WHO	Technical advice
The World Bank	Financial resources

resources of member organizations as needed and sharing in the costs of the secretariat. The primary role of each organization is outlined in Table 6.7. By defining clear roles like these in the First Mile and agreeing on a way to hold partners accountable for these roles, partnerships can avoid some of the conflicts that might otherwise arise.

In this chapter we have described the key elements a partnership needs to address in the First Mile. They are not the essence of what good partnerships accomplish, but they are the vehicles. If partners are able to hold open discussions about these elements—experiencing the inevitable conflicts, learning from them, and sustaining a collaborative spirit—they will gradually become a team. That is the real work of the First Mile.

The Task Force had that kind of experience. "On the whole," Bowles concludes, "the Task Force was a special place for the free exchange of ideas, information, and concerns related to the achievement of its goals." And that helped them accomplish what many had thought impossible: When they completed their Last Mile in 1990, the partnership had reached their goal of 80 percent immunization. They knew they had accomplished something really remarkable, and the partners we interviewed attribute that success to the close collaboration they achieved over the six years.[47]

In the end it is the growing sense of trust, an important part of a team's "social capital," that allows partners to develop that kind of high-level collaboration. One global health leader commented that global health partnerships are intrinsically unstable: the centripetal forces of a pressing need pull you together and the centrifugal forces of changes in governments, shifts in global health architecture, changes in membership, agendas of participating organizations, and funding issues pull you apart (as we mentioned in the earlier discussion on the PARTNERS project in Peru). As Ian Smith of WHO told us, "If there is no social capital, there will be enormous arguments about how to use the limited resources. If there is a good working relationship, people will do the right thing and put the money toward the cause in the best way possible."[48] Only when partners invest what some have called the "seed capital of trust" can they withstand these forces and successfully make the journey together.[49]

NOTES

1. Smith's comments are from a group discussion with the authors on May 8, 2008.
2. Bowles, *The Task Force for Child Survival and Development: Hope as Energy*, 2.
3. Ibid.
4. A. W. Claussen, McNamara's successor at the World Bank, was also included in this meeting.
5. Hinman, interview with the authors, December 7, 2004.
6. Hinman in ibid. These four stages of team development, long recognized by social scientists, are sometimes called "forming, storming, norming, and performing"— terms developed by McKinsey & Company to train its consultants. The "First Mile Toolkit" at the end of this book provides tools to help members agree on ground rules for meetings and guide facilitators to solve conflicts that may arise.
7. World Bank, *Addressing the Challenges of Globalization*.
8. Hardman's comments are from Coalitions and Collaboration in Global Health: A Symposium for Global Health Leaders, October 19–20, 2006.
9. Yip's comments are from a group discussion with the authors, May 8, 2008.
10. Berwick, interview with the authors, October 20, 2006.
11. Coll-Seck, interview with the authors, August 19, 2005.
12. Ibid.
13. A stakeholder analysis form is provided in the "First Mile Toolkit" at the end of the book. See Table 4.2 in Chapter 4 illustrating differences in perspective across organizations.
14. Villeneuve's comments are from an advisory group meeting with the authors, November 10–11, 2005.
15. Foege, e-mail to the authors, June 18, 2007.
16. Twum-Danso's comments are from an advisory group meeting with the authors, November 10–11, 2005.
17. Katzenbach and Smith, *Wisdom of Teams*, 48.
18. Ibid.

19. Berkley, interview with the authors, January 4, 2005.
20. Following the initial meetings, the heads of the member organizations sent their top deputies as representatives. During the first two years the representatives who attended regularly, according to meeting minutes, were Kenneth Warren (of the Rockefeller Foundation), Newton Bowles and Steve Joseph (of UNICEF), Rafe Henderson (of WHO), and Tony Measham and John North (of the World Bank). Bill Foege and Bill Watson (of the secretariat) also attended. Representatives from the Rockefeller Foundation attended conferences in the first three years and became active in quarterly meetings in the last three years of the effort.
21. Foege, interview with the authors, July 27, 2002.
22. Bowles, *The Task Force for Child Survival and Development: Hope as Energy*, 6–7.
23. The Warren quotation is in ibid., 7.
24. Caines, *Assessing the Impact of Global Health Partnerships*, 32.
25. Davidson, interview with the authors, November 5, 2002.
26. Bowles, *The Task Force for Child Survival and Development: Hope as Energy*, 7.
27. Such discussions can also lead to developing or refining the project charter—see the "First Mile Toolkit" at the back of this book.
28. Grant as quoted in Bowles, *The Task Force for Child Survival and Development: Hope as Energy*, 9.
29. Some partnerships have found it useful to test whether a goal is shared by doing a comparison of members' goals to the stated goal of the partnership (see the "First Mile Toolkit" at the back of the book).
30. Bill & Melinda Gates Foundation, *Developing Successful Global Health Alliances*.
31. Sharon Kagan's *United We Stand* (New York: Teachers College Press, 1991) refers to this type of governance as the "wheel."
32. Hinman, interview with the authors, October 15, 2004.
33. Bowles, *The Task Force for Child Survival and Development: Hope as Energy*, 3.
34. Foege, interview with the authors, August 16, 2004.
35. See the "First Mile Toolkit" at the back of this book.
36. Hinman, interview with the authors, October 15, 2004.
37. Katzenbach and Smith, *Wisdom of Teams*, 47.
38. Bowles, *The Task Force for Child Survival and Development: Hope as Energy*, 3.
39. Ibid., 16.
40. Ibid.
41. Foege, interview with the authors, July 26, 2002.
42. The "First Mile Toolkit" at the back of this book provides partnerships with worksheets they can use for discussing threats and opportunities, ranking opportunities, developing a strategy statement, and determining key activities, which can later be developed into a work plan.
43. Ross, interview with the authors, January 6, 2005.
44. Coll-Seck, interview with the authors, August 19, 2005.
45. Ibid.

46. Heymann's comments are from Coalitions and Collaboration in Global Health: A Symposium for Global Health Leaders, October 19–20, 2006.
47. The Task Force for Child Survival adopted additional goals and began a new journey in the following years, with new members participating.
48. Smith, interview with the authors, February 7, 2005.
49. The phrase "seed capital of trust" was drawn from Austin, Reficco, and Berger, *Social Partnering in Latin America*.

Discipline and Flexibility in Management

Jim Curran, the photographer who joined a group of climbers on K2, describes what it felt like to leave base camp and begin his journey up the mountain: "Would so many people moving up and down the mountain work out for good or bad? If harmony and co-operation prevailed, there could be a formidable collection of strong climbers breaking and maintaining trail which, after the bad weather, would be a more than normally arduous business higher up. But rivalry and discord could create a modern day Tower of Babel and the whole random collection of men and women striving for K2's summit might defeat themselves without any help at all from the mountain."[1] He might just as easily have been describing the challenges that lie ahead as a global health partnership begins its Journey.

This chapter and the next one break those challenges into management and leadership issues. While management is often considered a form of leadership, the separation into the two topics gives us a useful way to approach the issues, with "management" covering operational topics and "leadership" covering roles individuals can play to help the partners become an open, collaborative team that performs at a high level. This chapter focuses on the management challenges.

In the past few years global health leaders have increasingly pointed to the need for better management of projects. A report published by the Bill & Melinda Gates Foundation in 2002 gently prodded partnerships: "As our research has shown, a more disciplined approach to structuring and managing these alliances can lead to even greater impact from the limited resources that are available."[2] Bill Foege, who depended on Bill Watson for management of the Task Force for Child Survival, put the issues in perspective: "Early global health work looked to the skills of medical practitioners. . . . It is now apparent that the skills of planning, developing surveillance systems, analyzing data, using epidemiological findings, organizing logistics systems, delivering products, and evaluating results are even more important than medical or scientific skills. Increasingly, the field looks to problem solvers, managers, and people who know how to get things done."[3] For these reasons Foege concludes that "the lack of management skills appears to be the single most important barrier to improving health throughout the world."[4]

While the lack of management skills may be the greatest barrier, other circumstances combine with it to make the management task of global health projects daunting. These include the nature of projects, medical issues, in-country conditions, and the composition of the team.

The nature of projects:

- These projects are start-ups, without the benefit of a parent organization, established command-and-control, or incentives that motivate teams.
- Grants are usually short-term, so partners lack incentives to plan far in advance.
- Dramatic scale-up is often required, introducing major complexity for implementers.

Medical issues:

- Medical challenges arise on virtually every project.
- Interventions have evolved from an era of simple immunizations and treatments to today's highly complex interventions and long-term treatments.

In-country conditions:

- The social and economic conditions in the populations being served create a constant need to adjust strategies and tactics.
- In-country management capacity is often lacking.
- Projects are often conducted in environments of political and budgetary instability.

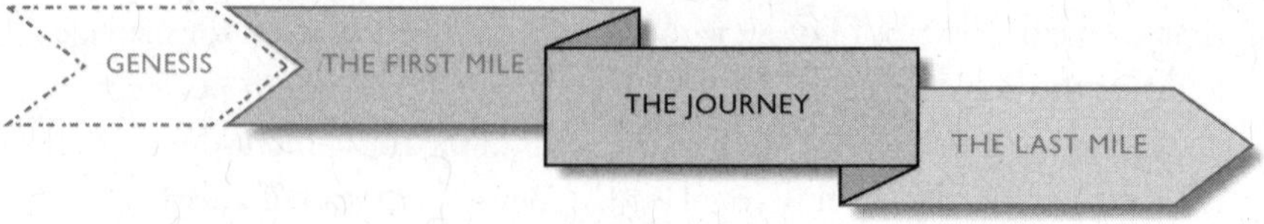

GENESIS | THE FIRST MILE | THE JOURNEY | THE LAST MILE

Key elements: Discipline and flexibility in management
• Applying discipline in research and planning
• Developing a considered approach to launching,
  measuring, and communicating
• Continuously engaging partners in problem-solving
• Revising the operating plan, based on learning

FIGURE 7.1   Partnership Pathway: The Journey. **Each partnership needs to invest time and effort to agreeing on the processes critical to meeting its goal and on ways to bring both discipline and flexibility to those processes.**

The composition of the team:

· Because teams typically involve agencies that compete for funding, members often have competing agendas.

· As Foege has pointed out, public health professionals often lack management skills; they are sometimes better at writing grants than translating plans into action.

These challenging circumstances constantly divert the energies of partners.

Given these inherent difficulties, how can partners manage global health projects effectively? In our research for this book, it became clear that partnerships need to create more discipline in their operating processes. In fact, in many areas of public health the business processes required to implement programs have never been clearly defined and widely agreed on. While the business community has developed a common base of knowledge and tools for such processes as sourcing raw materials or talent; developing products and services; marketing and distributing those products and services; and communicating the value of them to potential customers, the global health community lacks a comparable base of knowledge and tools. Given this reality, each partnership needs to invest time and effort to agree on the processes that are critical to meeting its goal and identify ways to bring discipline to those processes.[5]

At the same time, partnerships have to remain flexible to respond to changes in the environment. The best form of management for global health teams involves both discipline and flexibility. By using greater discipline in putting basic processes in place but relying on principles rather than a rule book in carrying them out, a partnership can respond to accumulating knowledge and to changing aspects of the project environment (social, political, and technological). This chapter describes how partnerships have used the following management processes and draws from their experiences some principles for applying these processes (Figure 7.1).

APPLYING DISCIPLINE IN RESEARCH AND PLANNING

In our research we heard complaints about excessive planning in global health, but we found that the problem was not excessive planning but *time wasted* in poor planning. The discipline of carrying out research and planning processes is critical, as Bill Foege stresses: "We need the same constant attention that is absolutely expected in the business community, with a focus on developing objectives, working out strategies for reaching those objectives, organizing all components of a program to pursue the strategy, pushing for continuous quality improvement, and developing the ability to measure both process and outcome goals for constant midcourse corrections."[6] The analysis of several partnerships helped us identify some useful principles to guide the partners' work in research and planning processes (Table 7.1).

The Research Process
The research process needs to help the partners determine the best approach in each geographic or population area for achieving their goal. To understand the scope of the problem and factors relating to it, the research may involve discussion with local communities, collection of data, and discussions with decision makers. As Nils Daulaire, the president and CEO of the Global Health Council, says, "Effective intervention begins with understanding the true nature of the problem, and the reality of ill health is that it is not just a biological issue but also a social issue in both its roots and its effects. Therefore, the first obligation of listening must be to focus on those most affected."[7]

The research should also involve understanding the point of view of key

TABLE 7.1 Principles for research and planning processes

Processes	Principles
Research	Involve local communities to identify social factors and political influencers
	Establish an early relationship with key influencers (including those responsible for budget decisions)
	Feedback research into the planning process
Planning	Agree on supporting strategies (such as the initiatives needed to carry out a surveillance and containment strategy)
	Build project plan around those strategies (plus a rigorous plan for evaluating progress)
	Connect planning to research by participating in multicenter prospective research on the interventions

influencers. Seth Berkley, the president of the International AIDS Vaccine Initative (IAVI), recalls a lesson he learned in South Africa:

> One of IAVI's great mistakes was not putting a person in South Africa and establishing a formal relationship. . . . South Africa was critical to our success. Nelson Mandela's physician advised the government to create SAAVI [South African AIDS Vaccine Initiative]. The SAAVI group didn't work out well and was disbanded. Because we didn't go there in the beginning, we lost an opportunity for working well with South Africa. We just didn't work hard enough at aligning interests.[8]

Among the key influencers IAVI and other partnerships need to understand are those responsible for budget decisions. In-country funding by the government is likely to be unstable unless the partnership can influence the next layer up from the ministry of health or educate those who can do so, such as doctors and nurses.

Finally, whenever possible, partners should participate in prospective research on the intervention outcomes. This research itself offers another chance at collaboration because research on scaling up and delivering interventions often requires the participation of multiple partners at many different centers. Global health projects tend to have an emergent quality because so much is unknown at the beginning. A disciplined research process narrows the uncertainties and gives the team a better sense of the challenges and opportunities they face.[9]

The Planning Process

With research completed, a partnership also needs to bring discipline and flexibility to its planning process. The overall strategy developed in the First Mile of the project will probably define the geographies to be served and how the partnership will approach the issues (such as the surveillance-and-containment strategy for the 1973–1975 smallpox efforts in India). But partners also need to define supporting strategies, such as strategies for acquiring and distributing drugs and delivering them to targeted populations.[10]

One partnership's experience with river blindness provides a good example. This partnership wrestled with how to deliver Mectizan in the area they were serving—Central Africa. Earlier in the book we described the context in which this partnership (the African Program for Onchocerciasis Control, APOC) began its work. In West Africa, where the disease had been most intense, the Onchocerciasis Control Program (OCP) had eliminated 80 percent of cases. The focus then turned in 1995 to Central Africa, where APOC began the battle to rid this area of river blindness as a public health problem by 2010.[11] Delivery of drugs was a crucial issue in planning how to achieve this goal.

Since the project covered the entire area of Central Africa, it had to be managed differently than the West Africa program.[12] "The whole project could have failed if we had rushed ahead before we understood the challenges of delivering so simple a product," recalls Raymond Gilmartin, then CEO of Merck.[13]

For example, APOC had to plan a new drug distribution strategy when it tried to extend its river blindness program into Sudan in the late 1990s, amid civil war. With the north and south of the country at war, the partners devised an unusual go-around. In a 2006 interview Bjorn Thylefors, the former director of the Mectizan Donation Program, recalls: "They agreed to establish a coordinating body for NGDOs [nongovernmental development organizations] in Nairobi for both the north and the south. It was expensive to get from Nairobi to southern Sudan, but it was a success under very difficult circumstances. The arrangement was acceptable to both north and south as long as it was transparent and fair to both sides. . . . When civil conflict exists, you have to establish a mechanism outside the government, but you have to find a way to support government policy at the same time."[14]

Although this distribution planning allowed APOC to succeed in Sudan, it would not be the last time the partnership had to reinvent its approach to distribution.

Once a partnership agrees on the right supporting strategies, it's important to turn them into a project plan with clear activities and ways to evaluate the progress of those activities.[15] At this point partners can see what responsibilities they may want to tackle, especially if organizational roles have not been determined in the First Mile. Without a clear operating plan and defined responsibilities, meetings can become a "group grope," in the words of one leader.

DEVELOPING A CONSIDERED APPROACH TO LAUNCHING THE PROGRAM, MEASURING PROGRESS, AND COMMUNICATING PROGRESS

Generally, global health partnerships have been quite successful at getting projects launched, particularly intervention projects. They have not, however, been as good at measuring progress and communicating with stakeholders. All three processes require a considered approach (Table 7.2).

Launching the Program

In launching the program, a key challenge is overcoming turf issues and creating impetus behind the effort. Several principles seem to help: (1) securing high-level backing, (2) supporting early adopters in their efforts to move the program forward in their countries or venues until it gains broader support, and (3) tapping community members to take advantage of their insights and build their skills for other public health projects.

For example, as the APOC partnership launched efforts in other regions, the pressing issue was not civil war (as in the Sudan), but simply finding enough people to do the job. Gilmartin recalls: "It almost did fail when we sought to manage Mectizan with roaming mobile teams—not a fea-

TABLE 7.2   Principles for launching, measuring progress,
and communicating

Processes	Principles
Launching	Tap community volunteers
	Secure high-level commitment and engagement
	Support early adopters
Measuring progress	Whenever possible, measure impact, not simply input or output
	Include sustainability indicators, such as donor satisfaction and funding commitments
Communicating with key stakeholders	Explicitly consider the attitudes of each stakeholder group before developing a communications plan
	Share credit

sible approach for covering thirty-three countries over fifteen years."[16] The partners realized they needed to tap community volunteers to administer treatment, and they developed a way to identify volunteers in each area and train them. Thylefors explains how APOC developed its new approach to delivering Mectizan:

> NGDOs got involved and we had a lot of discussions. Some people were negative about getting NGDOs involved, but they gradually learned to respect them, and we were fortunate that we had NGDOs that were committed for the long term. They realized we couldn't go on having boundaries and small teams, so they started community-based programs.
>
> [In these community-based programs, APOC made an important discovery]: The community got so educated that after a few years, realizing they would need many years of regular treatment, they wanted to take part in organizing for the next dose of Mectizan. That's when the Special Program for Research and Training in Tropical Diseases (TDR) got the idea to see if the villages could do it themselves. They did several studies that showed that villages could do it with minimal support. They selected people they trusted in the communities and gave them training.[17]

Community-directed treatment became the delivery strategy for APOC. With communities providing resources to conduct treatments, APOC and its subteams could turn their attention to measuring progress and refining treatment.

This experience taught project leaders a principle for launching programs that is making its way across global health efforts: community volunteers are a critical resource. The other two principles came from other partnerships—securing high-level engagement as well as community engagement, and supporting leaders who are early adopters.

Measuring Progress

The second important process at this stage is measuring progress effectively, a major lever for improving global health projects. One of the breakout sessions at an advisory group meeting for this book reported that: "People show up at a meeting cold all the time in global health, without thinking about what needs to happen in that meeting. They shoot from the hip in making decisions. That's permissible because nobody is checking the targets. Without profit and sales as indicators, as you have in business, the indicators are fuzzy." Rafe Henderson, formerly an assistant director-general of WHO, also stressed the importance of measurement: "If you can't evaluate your progress and results, it's very hard to hold a coalition together. You need to set clear objectives and monitor them to have a successful coalition."[18]

In recent years the World Bank and major foundations and coalitions have explored ways to improve measurement, and two principles have emerged: (1) whenever possible, measure impact, not simply input or output; and (2) include sustainability indicators, such as donor satisfaction and funding commitments. Regarding the first principle, no common definitions exist

> "Partnerships have clear goals because donors require it. Unfortunately, failure on those goals is a very common practice. They often set up very clear goals and communicate them but because of poor implementation, some of these projects don't have an impact on anyone."
>
> JIM KIM, Chair, Department of Social Medicine, Harvard Medical School, November 16, 2004, interview

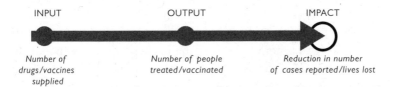

INPUT	OUTPUT	IMPACT
Number of drugs/vaccines supplied	*Number of people treated/vaccinated*	*Reduction in number of cases reported/lives lost*

FIGURE 7.2   Examples of measurements. **Teams need to measure clear progress toward the goal, not merely activities.**

across global health for the terms "input," "output," and "impact." In fact, under the general definition of the word "impact," both inputs and outputs could be considered impacts. It's useful, however, for teams to think of inputs as resources the partnership provides, outputs as people or communities receiving those resources, and impacts as changes in health or related breakthroughs linked to the goal. The semantics aren't really important as long as the team is measuring clear progress toward the goal and not merely measuring activities (Figure 7.2).

The second principle—including such sustainability indicators as donor satisfaction and funding commitments—keeps the partners alert to risks that funding may be discontinued.

Obstacles stand in the way of following these principles, however. One obstacle in developing countries is the lack of strong surveillance and monitoring systems. Until such systems improve, partnerships have to rely on measures of input or output for such populations. Another obstacle for some efforts is the length of time before impact can be determined. For example, with the launch of the Guinea Worm Eradication effort, it was difficult to measure impact because of the yearlong incubation period, so the partners had to start with measurements of input or output. Don Hopkins, vice president of Health Programs at the Carter Center, explains:

> In smallpox it was possible to show effectiveness after two weeks, an almost immediate impact. However, in guinea worm at least they could measure whether the four interventions were in place and show whether they covered all of the endemic villages with one or more of the effective interventions. They took these measurements monthly and compared them to progress in the same month the previous year.[19]

This yearly comparison of process helped them gauge the likely impact of current efforts and calibrate, as needed. Ideally, partners should use a balanced scorecard, not only measuring impact on targeted populations, but also including such sustainability indicators as satisfaction of donor expectations, funding commitments, and overall effectiveness.[20]

Communicating Progress

The third process important at this stage is communicating with key stakeholders about the issues of concern to them. The first principle for being able to do so is to explicitly consider the attitudes of each stakeholder group before completing a communication plan. For example, if stakeholders are skeptical about an intervention, early communication of progress is critical. Bill Foege recalls the importance of communicating success during the smallpox eradication effort in India:

> Forty years ago people believed that if you mess with culture, culture would always win. However, some cultural issues will disappear in the face of information. For example, in India they once believed in the smallpox goddess and thought it was a blessing for a person to get smallpox. However, when it became apparent that parents could do something to help their child, they changed and wanted to protect their children against the disease. Knowledge is powerful in the face of culture.[21]

Through intensive efforts to communicate progress to the villages affected, the teams were able to develop the impetus needed to stop the spread of the disease.

The communication plan need not be a complicated sheaf of papers but a simple plan that identifies key stakeholder groups and the right channels and timing for reaching each group. Traditional channels, such as speeches,

> "We must keep reminding stakeholders that we are there to make life better in the villages. We do that by having indices of progress."
>
> DON HOPKINS, Vice president, Health Programs, Carter Center, September 20, 2005, interview

newsletters, or e-mail (where viable), should be part of the consideration, but in developing countries it's especially important to take local preferences into consideration. For example, as mentioned in an earlier chapter, an advocacy effort for HIV/AIDS in Botswana effectively communicated its messages through a television soap opera.

A second principle is to share credit for successes. At the 2006 symposium President Jimmy Carter explained why the Carter Center decided not to put its name on information about the progress of the Guinea Worm Eradication Program in Latin America. It simply put the name of the program itself on news releases so the country leaders could take pride in their progress. By sharing credit in ways like this, teams can encourage local leaders to remain involved in the project and participate in future public health efforts. As Don Berwick, CEO of the Institute for Healthcare Improvement, told us: "Credit is infinitely divisible."[22]

These three processes—launching the program, measuring progress, and communicating progress—make an enormous difference in getting the partnership off to a good start. Partners must take the time to develop a considered approach to each process.

CONTINUOUSLY ENGAGING PARTNERS IN PROBLEM SOLVING

The processes we've described so far are needed in any global health project. The next key process—continuous engagement of the partners in problem solving—is relevant primarily for partnerships that are trying to develop into close collaborations. Because the partners may be preoccupied with responsibilities in their own organizations, we recommend two supporting processes to keep all partners involved in the problem solving that needs to

"The factors that have impeded momentum for alliances have been management issues, such as performance evaluation, clear and open communications, and a plan for sustaining funding."

ANIL SONI, Director of pharmaceutical services, Clinton Foundation HIV/AIDS Initiative, July 22, 2002, interview

TABLE 7.3   Principles for engaging partners in problem solving

Process	Principles
Holding productive meetings	Send materials in advance
	Shape agendas around issues, not reports
Communicating frequently with partners	Decide as a group on the best method (what, how, and when) for partner communications
	Seek partner feedback on new discoveries and on progress and openly discuss failures to learn from them
	If partners have difficulty working together, consider special mechanisms, such as an interagency coordinator

take place throughout program implementation. These include holding productive meetings and communicating frequently with partners (Table 7.3).

Holding Productive Meetings

The leaders we interviewed described the sense across global health that meetings are often a waste of time because little planning goes into them. One of the simplest ways to improve partner engagement is to hold meetings that focus on problem solving and decision making, not on reporting. A kickoff meeting of the Public Health Informatics Institute is a case in point.

> During the anthrax scares of 2001–2002 public health labs across the United States were overwhelmed by an avalanche of white-powder specimens that had to be examined for anthrax spores. Many labs were still using pen and paper to record information about the specimens, test procedures, and record results. When bio-preparedness funds became available, one of the first things many lab directors wanted was an improved information system.
>
> David Ross of the Public Health Informatics Institute proposed that the labs leverage their resources by working together to define the information needed. Although skeptical that the needs of their individual labs could be met by such a system, sixteen state and local lab directors attended the kickoff. Ross recalls an awkward moment during that meeting: "When the lab directors came to the kickoff meeting, we had a set agenda and slides

that went over the project in detail so we could sell them on the concept. Someone actually stood up the first morning and said this was a waste of time because we already had the commitment of the attendees."[23] Ross quickly changed course from presentation mode to problem solving and involved the directors in a discussion of the problem they were all concerned about—how to develop a system that would help them process all the samples of white powder flooding their labs.

Ross's willingness to shift the meeting agenda to problem solving gave participants the chance to learn from all the ideas in the room during that initial meeting, and the partnership took on a new tone. Much to the surprise of the lab directors, they found that approximately 85 percent of what they did was the same—including registering specimens, processing them, ordering reagents, disposing of biological wastes, and reporting results. Within six months they had developed a detailed list of common requirements for their information systems. Several states subsequently worked with vendors to develop the software.

Don Berwick also had an experience that required a change in agenda. He told us the story of a meeting his institute had organized in Bellagio, Italy, to examine the need for better approaches to defining, assessing, assuring, and improving the quality of health care in developing nations. He and his cochairs intended to promote the idea of an international "commission" to report on that need. They had prepared carefully to present an approach they felt was comprehensive, efficient, and effective. Instead, they were startled by the reaction they got from the participants from developing countries, the people they came to "teach." "Your proposal is simply wrong," they told him. "This plan might work for *you*, but it definitely won't work for *us*."[24]

All the preparatory work they had done was put aside, and Berwick and his team just listened. After a brief period of disorientation, they started to realize that the messages they were getting were clear, consistent, logical, and progressive. The more they listened, the more they learned, and they quickly began to reengage with the group on new terms toward a fresh, and much better, plan. The developing country representatives volunteered that it was rare in their experience to have such a plan (offered by would-be teachers from the North) dropped and redesigned based on their reactions. Berwick's team was equally impressed: "The amazing thing is that we came out with a much stronger approach than we ever would have dreamed of. For all of us it was a startling but priceless experience."[25]

The most important principles for focusing partner meetings on problem solving are to send materials in advance and base the agenda on issues, not reports. The agenda issues should be the most important ones facing the partnership. Alan Hinman, facilitator of the PARTNERS project in its early days, recalls: "One of the problems is that we all fell into the trap of the urgent driving out the important. Weekly videoconferences were almost exclusively dedicated to immediate problems. We should have focused more on the end result rather than the alligator chewing around our ankles."[26]

Communicating Frequently with Partners

Between meetings it's also essential to maintain frequent and transparent communication among partners so the partnership remains cohesive. Many partnerships never decide explicitly how and when they would like to receive information on the project. One partner may pass along information to another partner informally, while other partners remain in the dark. Eventually that kind of situation leads to distrust. The first principle for communicating with partners is to decide as a group *what* information the partners would like to receive, *how*, and *when*. Jim Kim of Partners in Health points out that the "how" is critical: "Personal relationships are very important in global collaboration. Therefore face-to-face meetings are the most effective ways to communicate. Videoconferencing is the next best form of communication, and then the phone, and the least favored form of communication is e-mail."[27]

A second principle that supports good communication between partners is asking members to provide individual feedback on the project. The feedback process can be as informal as a discussion or can take the form of a survey.[28] For example, a subteam of APOC—the National Onchocerciasis Task Force, consisting of national and international NGOs—meets monthly in

> "We also know that clear and frequent communication is the lifeline of any collaboration. For starters, good communication is vital to the building of the personal relationships from which trust emanates."
>
> JAMES E. AUSTIN et al., *Social Partnering in Latin America*

TABLE 7.4 Principles for revising the operating plan, based on learning

Process	Principles
Revising the plan	Establish a shortfall team
	Review shortfalls, to learn from mistakes
	Incorporate those lessons into operating-plan revisions

each country being served, with a national coordinator from the ministry of health who calls the meeting. Members update each other on the planned treatments, the need for tablets, and problems they are running into in a very down-to-earth way, according to Thylefors.[29] This communication approach helps keep the treatment programs moving forward.

A third principle for communicating with partners is to invest in a mechanism to improve understanding if it becomes clear that some of the partners have difficulty working together. Carol Pandak, a program manager with Rotary International, describes how the Global Polio Eradication Initiative handled such an issue in recent years: "They hired an interagency coordinator. . . . The position is paid for by several of the partners and his job is to organize partners. . . . His position is housed at WHO, and he spends one week per month at UNICEF. [Many of the issues are between WHO and UNICEF.] . . . He comes to Rotary, as needed, once every couple of months to get deep into Rotary culture."[30]

According to Pandak, this arrangement has made things run smoother. Even so, Pandak wishes for more frankness from Rotary's partners when the larger partnership group meets. "I would like to hear the realistic description of what is going on," she says. "Sometimes they seem to censor themselves because Rotary is a major donor to the initiative, even though we have committed to give the money until it's over."[31] As Pandak suggests, good communication between partners requires honesty and transparency. These three principles can help partnerships achieve that.

REVISING THE OPERATING PLAN, BASED ON LEARNING

Finally, partnerships need a process for digesting and incorporating what they learn into their operating plan, as APOC did with its community-directed treatment strategy. Most partnerships have every intention of learning from mistakes, but few establish a process to make sure that it takes place (Table 7.4).

To make sure the team learns from mistakes, it's important to establish a shortfall team that is activated by any failure to reach a milestone. As Nils Daulaire comments, "Learning is not possible without an honest assessment of failures and successes; every failure should be seen as an opportunity to assess, modify, and improve. Unfortunately, this rule is often abandoned in the efforts by some global health programs to attract and keep resources and the mistaken impression by some that leadership means 'never having to say you're sorry.'"[32]

To ensure that it learned from mistakes, the pharmaceutical company Merck established the Mectizan Expert Committee (MEC) when the first distribution programs were launched. This review team has been invaluable as the reach of APOC has extended farther across Central Africa. Thylefors explains:

> If there are unsatisfactory results, we take it back to the Mectizan Expert Committee and we decide on how things will be done with APOC. For example, when we had particular problems with Loa Loa in the Democratic Republic of Congo in 2004, we did that. Oncho can give you a lot of itching and dizziness, fatigue, headaches, and so on. But Loa Loa can probably create micro-emboli in your circulation system if not taken care of. One normally doesn't die from this, but we wanted to make sure there was no reason why there were so many side effects in some areas. MEC agreed with APOC to send an expert mission. We stopped the treatment, and we had four people in the area within six weeks to investigate it. The team found something else was causing the side effects: community workers had not been properly trained to do the on-the-ground work as carefully as needed.[33]

With that information, APOC quickly solved the problem. It revised its operating plan to include the needed training and moved forward once again with the implementation.

The practices APOC has followed have led to strong success in the areas it has served. "Today we look back and it's incredible how much you can achieve," says Thylefors. By 2002 the partnership was distributing Mectizan to more than thirty million people in thirty-three of the thirty-five countries where river blindness was endemic. By 2006, 117,000 communities were conducting their own treatment programs for more than 46 million people.[34] By the end of 2006 the partnership had decided to broaden its scope to include both lymphatic filariasis and other tropical diseases, to bring in additional partners, to expand its geographic spread to include the West African countries that had benefited from the OCP in earlier years, and to stretch its timeline to 2015.

APOC is one of many partnerships that have helped us frame the management approach described in this chapter, from preimplementation planning right up to the end of a project. In describing processes for each stage of program implementation, our intention is not to lay out a formula, but to begin the task of proposing useful management processes to improve the chance for success in global health projects. The principles, suggested by those who have participated in a variety of efforts, are intended as guidance, to help teams adapt readily to their own situations. As one global health leader told us, "We're always managing at the leading edge of how to do something." That takes both discipline and flexibility.

We look forward to the ideas other research teams and global health leaders will add to this approach, to help participants bring greater management discipline to global health. As many global health leaders have told us, good will is not enough to bring to a project. Increasingly, donors, partners, and recipients expect good management.

NOTES

1. Curran, *K2: Triumph and Tragedy*, 32.
2. Bill & Melinda Gates Foundation, *Developing Successful Global Health Alliances*, 6.
3. Foege in the preface to Foege et al., *Global Health Leadership and Management*, xxii.
4. Ibid., xxiii.
5. See the "Management Toolkit" in the back of this book for a worksheet to discuss management processes.
6. Foege in the preface to Foege et al., *Global Health Leadership and Management*, xxiv–xxv.
7. Nils Daulaire, "Leading for Success," in Foege et al., *Global Health Leadership and Management*, 219.
8. Berkley, interview with the authors, January 4, 2005.
9. See the "Problem Statement Worksheet" in the "Management Toolkit" at the back of this book.

10. See the "Opportunity Matrix" in the "Management Toolkit" at the back of this book.
11. APOC also sent tablets directly to West African countries, after the discontinuance of the OCP program.
12. As discussed in Chapter 4, in some areas drug distribution was further complicated by the need to distribute albendazole as well as Mectizan.
13. Gilmartin as quoted in Foege et al., *Global Health Leadership and Management*, 16.
14. Thylefors, interview with the authors, July 20, 2006.
15. See the "Consolidated Project Plan Template" in the "Management Toolkit" in the back of this book.
16. Gilmartin as quoted in Foege et al., *Global Health Leadership and Management*, 16.
17. Thylefors, interview with the authors, July 20, 2006.
18. Henderson, interview with the authors, October 20, 2004.
19. Hopkins, interview with the authors, September 20, 2005.
20. The concept of a balanced scorecard is captured in Kaplan and Norton, "Balanced Scorecard." See "Balanced Scorecard Worksheet" in the "Management Toolkit" at the back of this book.
21. Foege, interview with the authors, December 8, 2004.
22. Berwick, from Coalitions and Collaboration in Global Health: A Symposium for Global Health Leaders, held at the Carter Center on October 19–20, 2006. See the worksheets in the "Management Toolkit" for developing a communication plan and sharing credit.
23. Ross, interview with the authors, January 6, 2005.
24. Berwick, interview with the authors, October 20, 2006.
25. Ibid.
26. Hinman, interview with the authors, December 17, 2002.
27. Kim, interview with the authors, November 16, 2004.
28. See the "Partner Feedback: 10,000 Mile Checkup" worksheet in the "Management Toolkit" at the back of this book.
29. Thylefors, interview with the authors, July 20, 2006.
30. Pandak, interview with the authors, March 21, 2006.
31. Ibid.
32. Daulaire as quoted in Foege et al., *Global Health Leadership and Management*, 221.
33. Thylefors, interview with the authors, July 20, 2006.
34. Ibid. Amazigo, "Twenty Years of Mectizan Mass Treatment."

Chapter 8 | THE JOURNEY
Complementary Leadership Roles

Photographer Jim Curran's mountain-climbing team began to run into serious problems in their journey up the treacherous slopes of K2. Unfortunately, their leader was unable to guide them through these difficulties.

> "[His reluctance] was almost a matter of principle with him," Curran says, "for he always believed that leadership was unnecessary, just a word on a piece of paper to satisfy bureaucracy. But the fact was he didn't enjoy it and, because of that, wasn't very good at it."[1]

This attitude strikes a familiar chord in global health projects, where partners often focus on the intervention itself and pay little attention to leading the team.

Anyone who has participated in a global health partnership, however, knows how badly leadership is needed. As we described in Part 1 of this book, global health partnerships face extraordinary challenges. The dispersed authority across global health means these partnerships typically operate amid a confusing web of organizations; the nature of the disease or health threat often kicks up medical or political issues; and the cultural and social dynamics within a team and across the population being served are extremely complex. Like a mountain-climbing team, a global health

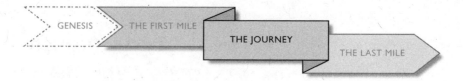

Key elements: Complementary leadership roles

- Filling critical team leadership roles
  - Convener
  - Visionary
  - Strategist
  - Team builder
- Serving external leadership roles
  - Advocate
  - Political influencer
  - Networker

FIGURE 8.1   Partnership Pathway: The Journey. **The most successful partnerships cover key team leadership roles and external leadership roles by allowing individuals to assume those roles in a complementary way.**

partnership brings an extremely diverse group of people into a highly unpredictable environment. Members are sorely in need of good leadership.

Given these challenges, we asked global health leaders about the kind of leadership needed for close collaboration. Their responses gave us an understanding of the critical team leadership roles during the Journey phase of a project (Figure 8.1), including the convener, the visionary, the strategist, and the team builder, and the critical external leadership roles, including the advocate, the political influencer, and the networker. But how could a team cover all these roles? As we examined partnerships and talked with those involved, it was clear that few of them managed to do it. The most successful partnerships covered these roles through complementary leadership rather than through a single strong individual.[2] As Kathy Cahill, a senior program officer for the Bill & Melinda Gates Foundation, said at our advisory board meeting, "Different skill sets are needed at different times. . . . Visionary people can attract followers, but they don't often have the right skill sets to carry out and implement the program."[3]

When partners begin to listen respectfully and openly share ideas, they develop an elasticity that allows one person to pull back and another to step forward, depending on the leadership needs of the moment. At such

TABLE 8.1 Team leadership roles

Team leadership role	Why important	Skills needed
Convener	Creates the "space" for open dialogue	Ability to suppress ego but keep driving for the goal
Visionary	Inspires partners with what can be accomplished	Ability to see the big picture and inspire others to pursue a goal
Strategist	Helps the partnership determine the value it provides	Rational thinking, with a background in framing strategic choices

moments, as individuals cede leadership to other partners, they build trust, and the bonds of close collaboration grow. Any individual who doesn't step back at such times risks losing the trust of the group. This chapter explores the leadership roles individuals can play in global health partnerships and how they can assume these roles in a complementary way. It draws on examples from the experience of the Global Road Safety Steering Committee (GRS SC), introduced in Chapter 4, but also includes lessons from other partnerships.

FILLING CRITICAL TEAM LEADERSHIP ROLES

Some of the leadership roles on a team, including the convener and visionary, are widely recognized, but the roles of the strategist and team builder often go unrecognized and unfilled (Table 8.1). The GRS SC is a good example of how these roles can play out in a partnership. The GRS SC was an informal partnership formed with a very specific purpose—to place global road safety on the agenda of the United Nations General Assembly. One of this book's coauthors, Mark Rosenberg, was involved in the partnership and provided some insights into how the leadership roles on the team developed.

While individuals and organizations across the globe had been advocating for road safety for many years and the World Bank had launched the Global

Road Safety Partnership in 1999, the GRS SC partnership was born out of the concerns of the Bone and Joint Decade (BJD).

Members of the BJD had a firsthand view of the rise in road-traffic injuries, and two of its orthopedic surgeons—Bruce Browner and Wahid Al Kharusi—conceived the idea of a conference on road safety at the UN. Rosenberg, who had been responsible for road-traffic injuries at the CDC and maintained this interest when he assumed leadership of the Task Force for Child Survival and Development, discussed the issue with Browner at a meeting convened by Michael Reich of Harvard. It quickly became clear that they shared a sense of urgency in addressing the problem, and they began to make plans for a partnership.

Funding for the partnership began to fall into place. Browner and Al Kharusi invited Rosenberg to speak on the subject at a meeting of the BJD in Rio in 2002. When the audience responded with strong concern and the BJD offered seed funding for a meeting at the United Nations, the three sensed the time was right for building political will. They contacted Kul Gautam at UNICEF to ask about the possibilities for funding an advocacy effort. Since a recent UNICEF report had highlighted the issue of road safety, Gautam was receptive and arranged for a small grant of $50,000 to support the partnership.

With guidance from the other leaders who had been advocating for a global effort, the three contacted critical stakeholder organizations, inviting them to participate. Eleven partners, including representatives from UNICEF, the UNDP, WHO, UNDESA [United Nations Department of Economic and Social Affairs], the BJD, the Task Force, the FIA Foundation, ASIRT [Association for Safe International Road Travel], the GRSP [Global Road Safety Partnership], and the Permanent Mission of the Sultanate of Oman (all of them individuals who were already working on the issue of road safety in their own organizations), held their first meeting in November 2002. Gradually others joined the effort. As Rosenberg recalls, "Everyone had doubts about how this effort would impact their own goals for road safety. Some were just willing to tolerate each other; some were willing to play an active role."

A small core group of active partners emerged in the Global Road Safety Steering Committee, and they filled the four team leadership roles: the convener, the visionary, the strategist, and the team builder.

The Convener

Whether a partnership is formally chartered or remains informal, someone needs to play the role of convener. Ideally this person not only sets up meetings but also facilitates them in a participative manner, setting a tone of open dialogue to create the "psychic space" that allows the group to work together successfully.[4] Bill Foege is widely mentioned as a model for the convener role in collaborative partnerships.

> Alan Hinman, who worked with Foege at the CDC, remembers: "He had the ability to submerge his own ego and not require recognition and he had a great sensitivity to others' thoughts and needs. [Foege's] gentle nature made it possible for him to be an effective facilitator. He established an atmosphere where people were not afraid to speak."[5]
>
> Rafe Henderson, then director of the Expanded Program for Immunization at WHO, echoes this sentiment: "Bill Foege brought a neutral middle ground to the Task Force. This meant that no agency was seen in competition with the other agencies." He added: "The role of neutral convener doesn't necessarily have to come from a separate group, but instead it is a specific quality in a leader who has a sense of openness to think and invent together."[6]

One of the most important steps Foege took in creating that environment was to talk privately with each member, learning what that member was passionate about. Once he found that out, he structured meetings to bring those interests to light.

It was Foege's ability to suppress his ego while still drawing on a deep well of determination that allowed the Task Force to drive forward and become a highly successful team. He had the characteristics of what author Jim Collins calls a "Level 5 leader." This type of leader, Collins says, "builds enduring greatness through a paradoxical blend of personal humility and professional will."[7] (This concept is reminiscent of Robert Greenleaf's description of servant leadership.[8])

With Foege as his role model and a small secretariat at the Task Force, Rosenberg served as the convener for the GRS SC. He worked to find common ground across the various purposes of the partnering organizations and helped the GRS SC build the cohesiveness to work together productively.

The lesson from this and other partnerships is for conveners to follow Foege's example—keep ego in check and create an environment that encourages partners to discuss and invent together. By tapping into members' intrinsic motivation and helping them understand each other, the convener can create a greater willingness to respectfully exchange ideas and begin to unleash the energy in the partnership.

The Visionary

One person on the team needs to paint a vision that inspires the partners and helps them maintain their focus on the goal. This role must be played by someone with a real passion for the issue and the ability to communicate that passion. Hinman describes a partnership that lacked that spirit: "In Atlanta we had a coalition of several world-class organizations. I was asked to serve as convener, but I wasn't the driving force behind the idea, and during my time on the coalition that leader never emerged.... The vision of what was possible together never appeared. Individual participants were doing things, but we weren't able to translate this into a group activity."[9]

We heard similar comments from other global health leaders about a number of coalitions. For the GRS SC "David Ward, Director General of the FIA Foundation, was the visionary," recalls Rosenberg, reflecting on the dynamics of the partnership.

> He had been waiting for leaders to step forward in road safety, and when we launched the effort, he was more than willing to participate. . . . He also brought with him an understanding of the scope of the issue and the life-changing impact safety efforts could bring. His informed vision of the impact of the partnership began to reassure the doubters on the team.
>
> At Ward's urging (and the strong support of BJD members), the partners agreed on their goal: to put the topic of road safety on the agenda of a United Nations Assembly meeting and generate a resolution supporting

---

"We need people who are facilitative, humble, and willing to share credit with the other partners and countries."

IAN SMITH, Adviser to the WHO director-general, November 10, 2005, advisory committee meeting

global efforts. Only then would they be able to attract regional and country funding for interventions.

Ward's presence on the Global Road Safety team filled a key need. As author Russell Linden says: "When partners believe that their work aims to change the world (even in some small way), and when they communicate that belief to others, their words and actions often instill the high stakes that help people cross boundaries and find common ground."[10]

The Strategist

A third essential team leadership role is strategist, someone with the ability to see the big picture and the small details simultaneously and articulate the possible pathways to achieving the goal. Fortunately for the GRS SC, Ward was able to think strategically as well as playing the visionary role. And Tony Bliss of the World Bank joined him in developing ideas for the team's strategy. "Tony had management experience, incredible energy, and a style that was non-turf-oriented and nonarrogant," says Rosenberg.

> These two partners worked together to develop viable strategic paths for the partnership. For example, when the World Bank decided to create a global funding facility for investment in road safety, the team discussed the possibility of developing an overall strategy for the facility. But they decided they lacked the money for developing a global strategy, and turf issues would make it difficult, in any case. Ward and Bliss recommended that the partners suggest action steps for the facility, avoiding the issue of a global strategy.

One or more members of a partnership need to lead strategic thinking in that way throughout a partnership's efforts.

The Team Builder

We heard more comments about the need for a team builder than any other role. This role involves helping the partners understand the various perspectives in the room and bridging those perspectives in a way that aligns all partners behind their central goal. To play this role without the benefit of traditional authority, one or more of the leaders on a global health partnership needs to have a style that is overarching and persuasive.

Susan Holck, director of general management at WHO, described the need for an overarching viewpoint early in our research for this book: "Collaboration takes place within a particular political context, a particular world context, and the 'cast of characters who are here now' context. It is not rational. It is about individuals working together or not, as the case may be. They all have their own issues, backgrounds, perspectives, and interests.... And their institutions also have all that, making it an incredibly complex mixture. We tend to underestimate all these factors in collaborating."[11]

Trying to create understanding requires a focused effort by a partner willing to play the role of team builder. The experience of the core team for the GRS SC, as they passed through the common phases of a collaborative team's development, illustrates the need for a team builder (Figure 8.2). Although the initial skepticism among the partners had subsided as Ward gave voice to their vision and Bliss joined him in laying out a practical strategy, the partners still had different views of how they should proceed. After the early meetings, when they had begun to recognize these differences in their individual approaches, they ran into conflict, which expressed itself as turf issues. Rosenberg explains:

> What happens in some organizations is they create a negative expectation of their people to work on teams. These organizations don't have enough money to really implement all the programs they would like to, so individuals get a distorted notion of power: the currency becomes power and recognition instead of achievement. So to rise in a bureaucracy you have to plant flags everywhere, claim authority. That shows how much you accomplished. It's the attitude of, "If we can't get rid of malaria, we can at least

"Getting partners to deliver on agreed commitments represents a challenge to many GHPs [global health partnerships]. This is partly explained by poor specification of responsibilities but more importantly by the horizontal and voluntary nature of partner relationships."

KAREN CAINES, Independent consultant, High Level Forum,
Assessing the Impact of Global Health Partnerships

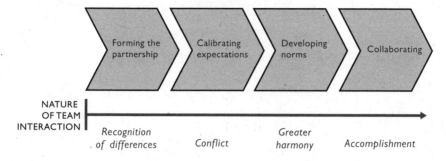

FIGURE 8.2   Phases of a collaboration team's development. **In becoming collaborative, teams pass through common phases.**

control all of those *working* on malaria." We had a member or two who got caught up in that. A leader has to think, "What can this person offer, and how can I get them to contribute that?"

Fortunately, when those members moved on to other projects, the remaining members were able to establish a good working relationship. Through a number of meetings during the next two years (over the phone and in person) the leadership pool expanded to include Fuad Mubarak Al-Hinai, UN ambassador from Oman and cousin to a member of BJD (who would assume an external leadership role). Through the goodwill of the partners, they developed the right chemistry, enjoyed open dialogues about the issues, and began to share a vision of how to address road safety.

Looking back on the experience, Rosenberg recognizes that, in addition to being the convener, he was trying to serve as the team builder, in conjunc-

"Technical skills don't necessarily equal emotional intelligence. The leadership skills we think of may not be in people who have the technical expertise. Also, since a lot of partnerships need to raise resources, these may be different skills from being a good collaborator."

SETH BERKLEY, President, International AIDS Vaccine Initative (IAVI), Coalitions and Collaboration in Global Health: A Symposium for Global Health Leaders, October 19–20, 2006

TABLE 8.2 Team leadership roles in the Global Road Safety
Steering Committee

Partner	Leadership roles
David Ward, FIA Foundation	Visionary
	Strategist
Mark Rosenberg, Task Force	Convener
	Team builder
Fuad Al-Hinai, UN Ambassador, Oman	Team builder
Tony Bliss, World Bank	Strategist

tion with Al-Hinai. But their partners often shared the team-building role with them. "While the secretariat had strengths," he says, "we also had weaknesses. If you're lucky, someone on the team will shore that up."

Viewing the GRS SC through the lens of these four team leadership roles, it's clear that members of the GRS SC beyond the core team contributed to all of these roles (Table 8.2). The partnership's gradual success also contributed to cohesiveness. As the GRS SC began to hold meetings at the United Nations, it became apparent they were making progress, and the partners who had been reluctant became less wary and more willing to share in the discussions.

Rosenberg recalls the interplay of these leadership roles as responsive rather than planned. "An informal partnership is fluid and chaotic at times, full of energy like a basketball game," he says. "Players have to be ready for the shot. And the key players may not be the ones you expect."

As the GRS SC partnership indicates, the right people to play the four team leadership roles are not always clear at the beginning. They often

> "I define 'collaboration' as caring about the people at the table as much as you do about your own perspective."
>
> **KATHY CAHILL**, Senior program officer, Bill & Melinda Gates Foundation,
> November 10, 2005, advisory group meeting

TABLE 8.3 External leadership roles

External leadership role	Why important	Skills needed
Advocate	Changing attitudes and behaviors	Ability to convey sincere passion for the cause
Political influencer	Tapping into the right people at the right time	Understanding of how decisions are made
		Ability to influence
Networker or connector	Generating wide support	Skills at maintaining a broad network of relationships

emerge as a kind of dance, one partner stepping back as another steps forward. As a partnership matures, the need for each role changes. Awa Marie Coll-Seck observed this dynamic in the Roll Back Malaria Partnership. "The challenge for leadership is to know when to step back or when to step forward," she has said. "It is not always evident when to do each one, but all partnerships must balance these roles."[12]

CRITICAL EXTERNAL LEADERSHIP ROLES

Successful partnerships also include external leadership roles (Table 8.3). Three closely related roles are needed on most partnerships: the advocate, the political influencer, and the networker.[13] (Note that all three roles require advocacy skills.) The road safety partnership provides a laboratory for understanding how these three external roles can develop on a team.

The Advocate

Every partnership has a need for someone to play an advocacy role, a passionate spokesperson who can champion the cause and sway others to support the project's goal.[14] In some cases advocacy is directed toward generating funds or services; in other cases the purpose is to bring NGOs and agencies on board. The GRS SC had an even broader advocacy task: to convince members of the UN General Assembly to support a resolution calling for road safety measures across the world.

While the members had begun to work together, aligned around their goal of holding a special UN meeting, "none of us had a realistic idea of how to bring this issue to the United Nations," Rosenberg admits. "It was a messy learning process, but we built momentum over time and we all benefited from Ambassador Al-Hinai's guidance." They started building awareness by holding a luncheon for UN ambassadors in January 2003, and in May of the same year, Alison Drayton of the UNDP briefed them on United Nations practices. Gradually they built social capital among the ambassadors and developed an understanding of how the UN operates.

Virtually every partner played the role of advocate at one time or another, but David Ward brought a special passion to this role. He was so enthusiastic and skilled that he succeeded in gaining the support of President Jacques Chiraq of France behind the idea of having WHO organize a World Health Day on the theme of road safety in Paris. Ward also brought his passion to meetings the other partners arranged with leaders the GRS SC wanted to influence.

In many cases, as Ward's example shows, the advocate may be the same partner who serves as the visionary.

The Political Influencer

Some partnerships have a need to influence government officials, whether the goal is funding, legislation, or behavioral change. Although the role of the political influencer is similar to the role of the advocate, the person who plays this role needs to have not only advocacy skills but also relationships among the targeted officials.

While Ward and others on the GRS SC had begun to generate broad support for placing road safety on the agenda of the General Assembly, a lot of one-on-one influencing still needed to take place among the UN ambassadors.

Two partners played roles as political influencers for the GRS SC. Ambassador Fuad Mubarak Al-Hinai was exactly the right kind of person to play the influencer role at the United Nations. He had been recruited to the partnership by his cousin, Wahid Al-Kharusi, who belonged to BJD's steering committee. Al-Hinai immediately provided access to other ambassadors and spent many hours consulting with the core team about how to approach UN officials. Tony Bliss also helped the team connect with stakeholders at the World Bank, which would ultimately provide a facility for funding road safety efforts.

Nearly every partnership needs people like Al-Hinai and Bliss who are well connected politically and willing to spend political capital to make things happen.

The Networker

The third external leadership role essential to global health partnerships is that of the networker. This role calls for a leader who has already developed a large web of relationships across multiple sectors. The networker is the one who can readily tap needed members for the partnership or open doors to talk with individuals who are key to carrying out a partnership's strategy. In many partnerships networking is focused on private industry or social organizations in the geography being served. In the case of the GRS SC, networking was particularly important among global health organizations, to ensure a united front for the ultimate goal of a UN General Assembly meeting focused on road safety.

Throughout the GRS SC's work, Rosenberg shared the role of the networker across the global health community with other members of the GRS SC. For example, his previous experience with various programs at UNICEF and WHO had given him contacts at those agencies, and in 2003 he spoke to J. W. Lee, director-general of WHO, gaining his support for the proposed World Health Day. Etienne Krug of WHO, also a member of the GRS SC, actively led World Health Day efforts at WHO and coordi-

"Among the distinctions between many health system leaders and transformational leaders is a breadth of perspective, comfort in bridging into adjacent policy domains, and the ability to influence based on broadly informed judgment rather than technical competence and credentials."

GARY L. FILERMAN, Professor, School of Nursing and Health Studies, Georgetown University

CLARENCE E. PEARSON, Former senior adviser, WHO,

"The Mandate: Transformational Leadership," *Critical Issues*

TABLE 8.4 External leadership roles in the Global Road Safety Steering Committee

Partner	Leadership role
David Ward, FIA Foundation	Advocate
Fuad Mubarak Al-Hinai, UN ambassador from Oman	Political influencer
Tony Bliss, World Bank	Political influencer
Rochelle Soble, ASIRT	Networker
Mark Rosenberg, Task Force	Networker
Etienne Krug, WHO	Networker
Wahid Al-Hinai, BJD	Networker

nated with UN agencies that were planning to celebrate World Health Day in 2004. That year he also coordinated the release of the landmark *World Report on Road Traffic Injury Prevention.*[15] Rochelle Sobel, director of ASIRT, brought invaluable support from U.S. politicians in Washington, D.C. Finally, Wahid Al-Kharusi used his global network through the BJD and an extraordinary network of health professionals in the world of sports medicine.

The team's success in building support across the global health community, Ward's passionate advocacy, and the targeted efforts of Al-Hinai and Bliss to influence political leaders took place simultaneously, with one partner networking among global health organizations while others exerted political influence with ambassadors and advocated with targeted individuals from all sectors (Table 8.4). The dynamic was different from the way they played the team leadership roles, with one partner stepping forward while another stepped back.

By playing the three external leadership roles simultaneously, the GRS SC partners were able to generate momentum and accelerate their team's progress. On April 14, 2004 (a week after World Health Day), the UN General Assembly held a special session focusing on road safety. In the daylong session, road safety advocates drove home their message to UN members. Karla Gonzalez, former vice minister for transport of Costa Rica, described the impact of an FIA-funded seat belt campaign in her country that catapulted usage from 24 percent to 82 percent in fourteen months. Ambassadors from Australia, Bangladesh, Ecuador, Egypt, Fiji, Iceland, Japan, Malaysia, and Thailand also came to the podium to address the seriousness of road-traffic injuries in their countries. At the end of the day, the General Assembly passed a resolution to improve road safety and designated WHO as coordinator for such efforts within the UN. The GRS SC sponsored a stakeholders forum the following day.

Within eighteen months of its formation, the GRS SC had accomplished its goal, an amazing feat in such a short time. They had prevailed through times of skepticism, conflict, and uncertainty about how to accomplish the task at hand. Following the successful UN meeting, the partners produced a report, *The Global Road Safety Crisis: We Should Do Much More.*[16]

The GRS SC concluded its work with the publication of that report. WHO assumed responsibility for coordinating UN agencies in efforts to pursue road safety, and the Global Road Safety Forum took the lead in organizing non-UN stakeholders.

As the experience of the GRS SC illustrates, leadership of a close collaboration in global health is unavoidably a team effort. That means any individual who plays a leadership role will have to give up some control so other partners can also lead. As Alan Hinman said in a speech at the CDC's Leadership Forum in 2006: "It is often said that there is no 'i' in 'team.' That is not really the case. The team is made up of a lot of 'i's who have given up some of their individuality to work together."

"By its very nature, the complexity of global health cannot effectively be addressed from a single vantage point, no matter how brilliant and committed the practitioner. And experience shows that all truly effective efforts to improve global health have been based on the thoughtful and coordinated work of teams."

NILS DAULAIRE, CEO, Global Health Council,
Quoted in *Assessing the Impact of Global Health Partnerships*

It is this sharing of leadership roles—this willingness to relinquish authority to others and give them the space to lead—that helps the partnership become an integrated team. When that happens, the possibilities for success open up and real problem solving takes place. Ed Baker, director for the North Carolina Institute for Public Health, says: "Over time I have come to the realization that the team precedes the idea. The best ideas emerge from within that team context."[17]

NOTES

1. Curran, *K2: Triumph and Tragedy*, 32.
2. While complementary leadership may be appropriate in most partnerships, it is usually not appropriate when a partnership is seriously threatened by external forces. At such times a single leader may need to step forward to play a more directive role.
3. Cahill's comments are from an advisory group meeting with the authors on November 11, 2005.
4. In the "Leadership Toolkit" at the back of this book, see the "Worksheet for Convener: Assuring Effective Meeting Management" to agree on participant roles for meetings.
5. Hinman, interview with the authors, December 7, 2004.
6. Henderson, interview with the authors, October 15, 2004.
7. Collins, *Good to Great and the Social Sectors*, 12.
8. Greenleaf, *Servant as Leader*.
9. Hinman, interview with the authors, December 17, 2002.
10. Linden, *Working across Boundaries*, 124.
11. Holck, interview with the authors, September 30, 2004.
12. Coll-Seck, interview with the authors, August 19, 2005. See the "Leadership Toolkit" at the back of this book for tools on team building and managing conflict.
13. In Chapter 6 we described institutional roles of partnering organizations. These external roles for individuals may reflect those institutional roles but typically go beyond them.
14. Gary L. Filerman and Clarence E. Pearson have pointed out the need for this skill, among others, in their article "The Mandate: Transformational Leadership."
15. WHO and World Bank, *World Report on Road Traffic Injury Prevention*.
16. The report was produced by the Task Force for Child Survival and Development in September 2004.
17. Baker, interview with the authors, January 6, 2005.

Chapter 9 | THE LAST MILE

The mountain climbers we've been following up the slopes of K2 struggled as the weather turned dangerous. Without strong leadership they had never become a real team, and conflicts began to surface. Photographer Jim Curran describes their state of mind:

> Our attempts on the North-West ridge had fizzled out with the knowledge that we had not even managed a summit bid. Given the weather and the weakened team, we have had no reason to reproach ourselves, let alone blame anyone, but by now no-one was particularly happy with themselves, or with others. It was 8th July and after six and a half weeks at Base Camp, we were having to start all over again.[1]

The team began to break up, and the attempt to reach the summit by the few who remained ended in failure and tragedy.

Researching the experience of global health partnerships, we found many of them had also become divisive and discouraged, and never completed their Journey. In contrast, those partnerships that found a way to work together and continued on the Journey reported a galvanizing moment when they realized the end was in sight—they would actually achieve the goal that had often seemed impossible.

When a team reaches this moment, they've entered their Last Mile, and it's a signal for them to think about their remaining work in a different way. Bill Foege's experience with the smallpox eradication program beautifully illustrates a team entering its Last Mile. He described his experience in an interview.

Earlier we described the impetus that came with new ways of delivering the smallpox vaccine. In 1967 that impetus made its way to India through the Intensified Smallpox Eradication Program, which used the freeze-dried vaccine. With the assistance of many outside organizations, Indian health officials first tried to control smallpox through mass immunization, but the country's size and enormous population, as well as the difficulty of reaching people in remote areas, frustrated their efforts. The number of smallpox cases climbed to 87,000, more than in any other country.

It was 1973 when Foege responded to a plea from WHO to assist with the immunization program in India, and he arrived with an innovative point of view about how to approach it. He had learned an important lesson in 1966, when a smallpox outbreak hit Biafra, Nigeria, on the eve of civil war. The conventional response would have been to vaccinate everyone, but that was impossible because of a shortage of vaccine. He directed his team to map the spread of the disease and to vaccinate people only in villages where smallpox had already appeared and in the immediately surrounding areas, containing the spread within the immunized ring. Four weeks after the first case had surfaced, no new cases were reported in eastern Nigeria. Foege and his team had devised the "containment" strategy that would eventually lead to global eradication.

Foege believed this containment strategy was the answer for India as well. Working directly with government leaders in Bihar, India's most impoverished state, and Uttar Pradesh, its most populous, he helped develop a sense of urgency for addressing the disease and mobilized funding support from industries that had been affected. He also convinced Indian health officials to shift from the unsuccessful mass-vaccination approach to the containment strategy. These efforts occurred before the era of formal partnerships and multiagency participation that would characterize the turn of the century. Instead, the program involved CDC staff members and district health officials and workers, who met every month and reported their progress.

With Bill Watson as his chief administrator, Foege developed informal partnerships with these groups in a large number of districts and invested a great deal of energy in building trust. For example, he knew success depended on motivating thousands of highly dispersed workers to map the incidence of the disease in more than 700,000 villages and quickly contain the threat. Putting his own life at risk, Foege carried millions of rupees in his briefcase and rode the trains across the country to ensure that health workers received their salaries. This dedication to building trust would later prove pivotal.

The darkest moment came on a Friday in May 1974, when eleven thousand cases were detected in Bihar, more in a week than had been reported in all of West Africa in an entire year. "Someone convinced the minister of health in Bihar that we needed to go back to mass vaccination," Foege recalls. "Otherwise he would seem powerless. Some say that power corrupts and absolute power corrupts absolutely but, to summarize the words of Paul Warnke, the most corrupting of all is the fear of loss of power."[2] Foege debated the issue with the minister of health: "I said that they had tried mass vaccination for 150 years and it hadn't worked. We had only tried the new strategy for seven months and we were asking for just one more month. The minister said, 'No, all thirty-one districts of Bihar have shown a continuing increase.'"[3]

At the district meeting the following Monday, the minister of health announced the decision to shift back to the old strategy. The group initially sat in stunned silence, then a dramatic scene unfolded. A young Indian physician from New Delhi rose and said, "I am just a poor villager and I don't know much, but I do know one thing: when I was growing up in the village, if someone's house caught on fire, we only put water on that person's house." The minister was startled, Foege recalls. "You could see he was wavering. Finally he said, 'This is so tough for me, but I am going to give you one more month.' We didn't know that day whether we would get over the hump. It turned out that it was a tipping point. The reported cases started dropping shortly after that, so the minister of health allowed us to continue."[4]

The same pattern occurred throughout the country, and by the end of 1974, Foege sensed victory over smallpox.

The eradication effort in India was in its Last Mile. When a partnership reaches the Last Mile and the goal is within grasp, it is tempting to go on autopilot. But we found that the teams in India and other real collaborations did exactly the opposite: they became more flexible and inventive,

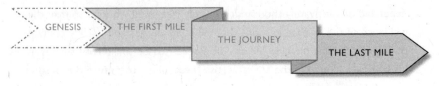

Key elements

- Adapting approach to sustain momentum
- Transferring control in a supportive way
- Capturing and communicating lessons learned
- Dissolving the partnership when the goal is achieved

FIGURE 9.1   Partnership Pathway: The Last Mile. **Instead of going on autopilot in the Last Mile, teams need to become more flexible and innovative in finding ways to reach their goal and complete their work.**

finding new ways to reach their goal and ensuring their task was fully completed. Their experiences provide lessons for other teams in dealing with the key elements of the Last Mile: adapting their approach to reach the last people affected by the disease/threat in a way that is practical, given the cost and effort per patient, transferring control in a supportive way and making sure the right people get the credit, capturing lessons learned and communicating them where they'll count, and dissolving the partnership when the goal has been achieved (Figure 9.1). In illustrating these lessons, we draw primarily from the efforts to eradicate smallpox in India and polio in the Americas.

ADAPTING THE APPROACH TO SUSTAIN MOMENTUM

The leaders of highly successful partnerships are absolutely determined to take the effort across the goal line. And to do that, they often find it necessary to adapt their approach—changing surveillance, stakeholder involvement, or strategy. As James Austin, professor emeritus at Harvard Business School, points out, "Sometimes there are unforeseen cultural difficulties, as in [the efforts to eradicate] polio. You need to know that can happen in the Last Mile." He adds, wryly: "The Last Mile may have to be an elastic measuring tape. You may see the finish line, but someone runs ahead of you to move it."[5]

The story of polio eradication in the Americas illustrates how one partnership evolved to reach its Last Mile and the changes it made at that point.

As described earlier in the book, when WHO declared victory over smallpox in 1980, the global health community began to anticipate the next possibility for eradication. Why not polio? After all, vaccines were available for this disease, too. These were exactly the thoughts of Ciro de Quadros, a Brazilian epidemiologist who headed the immunization program of the Pan American Health Organization (PAHO), the regional arm of WHO in the Americas. Starting in 1980, on two weekends he and his colleagues held National Immunization Days in Brazil, vaccinating about twenty million children under the age of five each weekend.

They were elated by the results. "Cases of polio dropped dramatically from an average of over one hundred to two hundred cases per month to fewer than twenty," he wrote in the 1997 book *Polio*.[6] Buoyed by these results, de Quadros urged the director of PAHO, Carlyle Guerra de Macedo, to take eradication across the Americas, and in 1985 PAHO boldly announced a goal of eradicating polio across the Americas. To plan the effort, de Quadros brought in Bill Foege, D. A. Henderson, Alan Hinman, and Jesus Kumate from Mexico, and João Batista Risi from Brazil, and they all supported his conviction that eradication was possible. Two years later, with funding commitments in place, several agencies formed a partnership to pursue that goal, the Inter-Agency Coordinating Committee (ICC) for Latin America and the Caribbean. It included representatives from PAHO, UNICEF, UNAID, the Inter-American Development Bank (IDB), Rotary International, and the Canadian Public Health Association.[7] This partnership met every three to six months to discuss issues and solve problems. An interagency committee was also formed in each country, chaired by the respective ministers of health.

In the first year one obstacle after another came up, recalls de Quadros.[8] "It was very difficult because every agency, every partner had a different agenda." For example, "USAID had strong objections to what they called a vertical approach or top-down campaign." WHO's director-general, Halfdan Mahler, also strenuously opposed the vertical nature of de Quadros' plan, believing it would detract from efforts to expand primary health care.[9] The lack of surveillance systems in many of the countries was also a problem, and civil unrest in El Salvador and Peru threatened to prevent immunization in those countries. De Quadros, whose office served as the secretariat, also had to build confidence among the leadership of the countries involved. "My first year," he says, "I spent a lot of time going to countries to put out the fires until we got everyone working harmoniously."

By the second year, however, the ICC had found ways to address these issues. Warring parties in El Salvador agreed to "days of tranquility" so children could be immunized, for instance. And Mahler and others realized that by offering primary care services as well as immunization on National Immunization Days across the region, they could actually strengthen primary care efforts. The mass immunization strategy proved to be powerful. In 1988 confirmed cases declined by 49 percent from a year earlier, and by July 1989, they had dropped 71 percent over the previous year. The disease was no longer evident in thirteen thousand districts, remaining active only in a thousand. The goal was in sight; the effort to rid the Americas of polio had entered its Last Mile.

In this partnership, as in other successful partnerships we researched, the partners approached the Last Mile with a willingness to be flexible in order to reach their goal. This flexibility was apparent in their surveillance efforts, increased involvement by local stakeholders, and even in their strategy.

Shifting the Approach to Surveillance

In the Last Mile the ICC dramatically improved surveillance, both by launching a comprehensive system and by shifting the focus of monitoring.

The computerized surveillance system, launched in 1989, involved a network of 22,000 health institutions that reported weekly on suspected cases. It would later be characterized as the most comprehensive surveillance system for human health that had ever existed in the hemisphere. Teams in the Americas (as in other regions of the world) also changed the focus of their surveillance in the Last Mile. The practice at the start of polio eradication programs was to monitor for flaccid paralysis because about half of such cases had historically been caused by polio. Teams would then divide by half to estimate the number of polio cases. As polio cases dropped, however, the percentage changed, and teams had to go beyond counting flaccid paralysis cases and actually conduct tests for the polio virus as part of their surveillance efforts. These changes were critical to achieving the goal.

In other partnerships focused on intervention, we also found that a change in approach to surveillance was often needed in the Last Mile as the number of cases declined. While increasing capabilities to conduct surveillance earlier in a partnership typically lead to detection of a greater number of cases (and assistance to more people), the number of cases detected drops as a partnership nears its goal. At this point partnerships have to work harder to find cases. For example, Don Hopkins, who was then a CDC representative to the Guinea Worm Eradication Program (GWEP), describes how GWEP shifted its approach to surveillance as the number of cases fell:

> In the beginning, GWEP focused on nations with heavy infestation of guinea worm. The partners faced pressures to invest in other diseases—for example, UNICEF pushed early on for GWEP to use resources for health issues other than guinea worm. But GWEP did not see their role as providing surveillance for villages that didn't have guinea worm.
>
> In the final stretch of eradication, that changed. Every case that turns up counts, but it doesn't make sense to have widespread surveillance aimed at a single disease at that point, even one aimed at eradication. In the end programs realized that other agencies were important because GWEP needed to be part of a broad-based surveillance system that would carry guinea worm surveillance. They pushed governments and other agencies to help finance broad-based, nationwide surveillance systems.[10]

This shift in approach to surveillance was very different from the shift in the polio eradication project in the Americas.

In the smallpox eradication effort in India, as mentioned in Chapter 3, the project team also shifted their surveillance strategy as the number of cases reported fell. To encourage the reporting of cases, they began to emphasize a system of rewards they had developed for the general public and for public health workers. The writer Elizabeth Etheridge describes this effort in *Sentinel for Health*:

> Beginning in October 1973, every village and every house in it were visited once a month. . . . In the village marketplaces, team members handed out

smallpox cards showing a picture of a smallpox victim and offering a $12.50 reward to anyone who reported a new case. Toward the end of the campaign, this tactic proved to be the most effective one in Foege's arsenal.[11]

At the time Foege worried that the surveillance was not as thorough as it needed to be, but in retrospect he believes it was good enough: "With a limited number of treatment teams, they could only cover a hundred villages at a time, and with the incentives, surveillance was good enough to keep those teams busy."[12] (The polio partnership in the Americas also used a reward system as the effort neared its end.) In the Last Mile of all these efforts, a key to sustaining momentum was the willingness of teams to substantially change their approach to surveillance.

Involving Local Stakeholders

Another way successful teams adapt to the needs of the Last Mile is to place greater emphasis on involving local stakeholders as the rollout extends to additional communities. For example, the efforts to control river blindness changed over time to increase the involvement of local stakeholders. Instead of sending mobile teams of experts to administer treatment, the partnership began to mobilize community workers.

To the extent that tasks change in the Last Mile (at a time when funding is running out), new partners and other resources from inside a country, as well as outside, may also be needed. James Austin put it this way: "You often need to mobilize resources for the final big push, just when funders think the problem is solved."[13]

Adapting Strategy

Successful partnerships (and the broader programs under which they may operate) are also alert to changes in the environment that may have strategy implications in the Last Mile. Don Hopkins recalls one such incident:

> I reviewed a report on another program that said one of the cardinal principles was to maintain their strategy. That was a danger signal, in my opinion. Any disease control program that goes in with the objective to preserve the strategy is flawed. It might be the best strategy now, but that doesn't mean it will remain the best strategy throughout the program. Smallpox changed from mass vaccination to case containment. Guinea

worm changed from a water-based strategy to a focus on health education and filters, along with water supply and Abate.[14]

Foege agrees with this assessment: "For me the model is to choose the objective and realize you are going to be changing strategy as you go forward."[15]

For example, in the polio eradication effort across the Americas the ICC shifted from a mass campaign strategy of National Immunization Days to a targeted strategy of containment in the communities where cases were reported; where coverage was low; or where overcrowding, poor sanitation, weak health-care infrastructure or heavy migration prevailed.[16] "Operation Mop-Up" focused intense efforts on these communities, sending teams house-to-house in two vaccination campaigns. These targeted efforts allowed the partnership to reach its goal, and in 1994 an internal commission declared that polio had been eradicated in the Americas. Like the polio effort, the other successful partnerships we examined were so determined to reach their goal that they readily shifted their strategy and tactics to get there, like water flowing around obstacles.

Those are some of the ways that partners we interviewed adapted their approach in the Last Mile, changing things as fundamental as surveillance, stakeholder involvement, and strategy, or simply being inventive in figuring out how to get past day-to-day barriers.

TRANSFERRING CONTROL AND GIVING CREDIT

In addition to adapting, successful partnerships begin to plan how they will transfer control of the project to regional and local leaders as soon as the team senses the Last Mile has begun. Eric Ottesen, director of the Lymphatic Filariasis Support Center at the Task Force for Child Survival and Development, advises that "as part of the exit strategy, you need to transfer control over revenue and ensure a revenue stream for sustaining the effort."[17]

> "Often the race is decided by how deep you can dig within yourself to take you across the finish line. You don't stop jogging two steps before."
>
> JAMES AUSTIN, Professor emeritus, Harvard Business School, Coalitions and Collaboration in Global Health: A Symposium for Global Health Leaders, October 19–20, 2006

Closely linked to the transfer of control is the need to give credit, both to in-country partners and to other partners on the project. Foege taught the global health community this lesson during the Last Mile of smallpox eradication in India.

> In less than two years the containment strategy had proven extremely successful in reducing the number of active smallpox outbreaks in India. By the end of 1974 it became clear to Foege that within the next several months the last active outbreak would be controlled. India was on the verge of an extraordinary achievement. At that time he notified his boss, David Sencer, the director of the CDC, that Foege and his family were returning home to Atlanta. Sencer asked Foege if he realized how important an achievement this would be in the history of global health, and counseled him not to come home before eradication was completed.
>
> Despite Sencer's protests, Foege left India before the disease was eradicated. He later explained the rationale: "I wanted Indian officials and public health workers to get the credit for the remarkable work they had done." Foege knew that recognition would motivate them to work hard in future health efforts.[18] In the spring of 1975 officials in India proudly announced that no cases of smallpox had been found.

Giving credit where it is due is not an unusual concept in global health. But a number of people we interviewed mentioned Foege's example of giving credit to in-country partners as an illustration of the extra effort needed to build capacity and relationships. In the words of Don Berwick, "Credit should be infinitely divisible."[19]

CAPTURING AND COMMUNICATING LESSONS LEARNED

Another important task at this final stage of the Partnership Pathway is to capture the lessons learned so other global health projects can benefit from that knowledge. Jim Kim of Partners in Health gives an example of an important lesson learned from treating multi-drug-resistant TB (MDR-TB):

> Insights from this project will be very helpful in shaping how we set up referral systems in developing countries for HIV treatment. We learned

that, to the extent possible, you should simplify and standardize as much as possible. With HIV treatment in developing countries, reaching scale requires at least some degree of simplification and standardization. We have been trying to provide workable guidelines for treatment for the 85 percent of patients who do just fine on first-line regimens. Those are people who get one pill in the morning and one in the evening and do just fine for three to five to seven years. Then as they go to second-line regimens, we have to have a good combination of second-line drugs and try to simplify again. Individual clinical management is important, but to reach as many people as we can, we have to find a way of extending the reach of physicians through nurses and community health workers. How do you organize health services in a way that keeps it simple when possible but can move to complex management when necessary? I think we came to some very good conclusions as to how to do that in MDR-TB.

People who designed the system for MDR-TB should sit down and talk about what we learned about this design and think about the implication for HIV treatment programs. You can't say DOT (Directly Observed Therapy) with the HIV community, but you can say "intensive adherent support." The lessons from DOTS (Directly Observed Therapy Short-course) and DOTS-Plus are absolutely critical in giving us the vision of where we ought to be in the next three to five years in HIV.[20]

Typically, such lessons learned are communicated in reports and articles, and the Internet has also become a means of determining and communicating these lessons. But Kim points out that the communication of lessons learned can take the form of workshops and conferences as well as publications.

Lucy Davidson, director of the suicide prevention program at the Task Force for Global Health, provides an example of how conferences can capture and communicate lessons learned. She describes a national conference on suicide prevention for 450 people in Reno, Nevada, that took place on October 17–18, 1998:

We asked the regional public health advisers to be the facilitators of the regional work groups, which were given the task of providing input and ranking ideas. The advisers were facilitating work they had never been thinking about or involved in, but the work groups were a mixture of clinicians, advocates, survivors, business, and community people—all of them individuals who really knew the issues. The regional public health advisers left there feeling that this work was very important—that it was definitely a public health issue and would have a public health response.[21]

By involving regional public health workers in capturing lessons learned, the suicide prevention program not only ended up with better plans, they also ended up with enthusiastic supporters. This lesson may be helpful in other projects that involve educating public health workers about the need for action in a particular health area. James Austin emphasizes the importance of capturing such lessons: "It's really important to reflect on why it worked or didn't work and what the implications are for going forward. We're engaged in a collective learning experience in the global health community."[22]

DISSOLVING THE PARTNERSHIP

One of the toughest decisions for a successful partnership is to disband when the work is finished, as Foege did with the smallpox eradication program in India. Especially in successful partnerships, members value the trust they have built and are reluctant to walk away. But trying to continue a partnership once its goal is met tends to create confusion and waste resources. The history of global health is footnoted with partnerships that tried unsuccessfully to continue past their declared goal. When this happens, an agency or organization can end up trying unsuccessfully to conduct its business through a set of subprime partnerships, which can be both costly and nonproductive. Our advisory group suggested that coalitions in

"In alliances it's rare that individual members stop doing things they were doing the day before. Unlike business, global health doesn't have 'creative destruction,' which happens when one company buys another."

MICHAEL CONWAY, Partner, Global Public Health Practice, McKinsey & Company, Coalitions and Collaboration in Global Health: A Symposium for Global Health Leaders, October 19–20, 2006

global health should be terminated when the project is over—or earlier if the project is just limping along.

As the examples in this chapter have illustrated, the Last Mile of a partnership is characterized by a number of contradictory forces. The partners must often work even more intensely to complete the effort at a time when their minds inevitably turn to their next projects. They must become more flexible just at the time when each step can change the outcome. But the greatest contradiction of all lies in the emotional downswing many feel just when the goal has been achieved.

D. A. Henderson, who had worked with Foege in India, remembers the sense of regret he felt once the effort had been completed and the World Health Assembly (WHA) announced the eradication of smallpox on May 8, 1980. "That was a defining moment," he recalls, "but it really was the end. It was what we had worked for, for years, but ironically it was also a kind of letdown. We were used to working in the field with so many wonderful people, sharing meals and sharing problems, sharing a real camaraderie, and developing deep friendships. We were like soldiers in the battlefield, but now the enemy was no more and we realized we would likely not see these people, these disease warriors, again. The joy was in the trip rather than in the arrival."[23]

NOTES

1. Curran, *K2: Triumph and Tragedy,* 86.
2. Opening remarks at Coalitions and Collaboration in Global Health: A Symposium for Global Health Leaders, the Carter Center, October 19, 2006. Paul Warnke served as assistant secretary of defense for international security affairs for President Lyndon B. Johnson and later as chief negotiator in strategic arms talks with the Soviet Union during the Carter administration.
3. Foege, interview with the authors, December 8, 2004.
4. Ibid.
5. Austin's comments are from Coalitions and Collaboration in Global Health: A Symposium for Global Health Leaders, the Carter Center, October 20, 2006.
6. De Quadros, "On toward Victory."
7. Individual representatives were Juan Agillar from UNICEF, Paula Feeney (followed by Carol Dabbs) from USAID, John Sever and Ted Trainer from Rotary International, and Edward Ragan from the Canadian Public Health Association. IDB delegated its representation to de Quadros of PAHO.

8. De Quadros, interview with the authors, October 23, 2007.

9. Fujimura, "Man Who Made Polio History," 2.

10. Hopkins, interview with the authors, September 20, 2005.

11. Etheridge, *Sentinel for Health.*

12. Foege's comments are from Coalitions and Collaboration in Global Health: A Symposium for Global Health Leaders, the Carter Center, October 19, 2006. .

13. Austin's comments are from Coalitions and Collaboration in Global Health: A Symposium for Global Health Leaders, the Carter Center, October 19, 2006.

14. Hopkins, interview with the authors, September 29, 2005.

15. Foege, interview with the authors, December 18, 2005.

16. Levine, *Millions Saved.*

17. Ottesen's comments are from an advisory group meeting with the authors, November 10–11, 2005.

18. Foege, interview with the authors, December 8, 2004.

19. Berwick's comments are from Coalitions and Collaboration in Global Health: A Symposium for Global Health Leaders, the Carter Center, October 19, 2006.

20. Kim, interview with the authors, July 7, 2005.

21. Davidson, interview with the authors, November 5, 2002.

22. Austin, interview with the authors, October 2006.

23. "Smallpox Eradication: Memories and Milestones," 5.

Chapter 10 | WAYS FOR DONORS TO ENCOURAGE COLLABORATION

Dramatic forces have swept through global health since the mid-1980s, shattering the architecture that had given shape to the field, multiplying the number of participating organizations, and increasing the expectation that recipient countries should participate in decision making. In this new environment individuals from every sector have voiced a need for working together more effectively and shared with us their lessons learned for achieving real collaboration. A pivotal force for ensuring these lessons are applied is the donor community—the global agencies, bilaterals, multilaterals, NGOs, foundations, and private-sector organizations that have made a commitment to global health. They have the power of the purse strings, the reach of multiple projects, and the stability to stay the course.

The role of Rotary International in the Global Polio Eradication Initiative (GPEI) is a good example of the central role donors can play. In the efforts to eradicate polio worldwide, Rotary International has been a sustained source of funding and an active partner for more than twenty-five years.

A call went out in the late 1970s to determine what big project Rotary could undertake for its seventy-fifth celebration. . . . Dr. John Sever suggested polio," recalls Carol Pandak, manager of PolioPlus for Rotary International.[1] It seemed an ideal project: an oral vaccine was available that could easily be administered, and the disease affected children from all walks of life, freeing it from social stigma and the barriers that might pose. The board of directors agreed, and Rotary (which had supported polio immunization since 1975) made a pivotal commitment to eradicate polio worldwide. They invited Albert Sabin, who had developed the oral vaccine, to speak at their 1985 convention, and his dramatic address riveted the membership and deepened their commitment.

One of the first challenges for Rotary and its partners was to generate the political will that would spur governments to provide resources. The early rumblings of success occurred in May 1988 at the United Nations, when the ministers of health of some of the world's largest countries led the effort to convince other nations that polio eradication was the right thing to pursue. Initially, global leaders resisted the idea of a program focusing on a single disease, since at the Alma Ata International Conference on Primary Health Care they had agreed that broader programs covering the spectrum of health issues were a more effective approach. But the success of Brazil's program (followed by the launch by the Pan American Health Organization [PAHO] of an eradication effort across the Americas) turned their thinking and led to an endorsement of eradication at the 1988 Talloires meeting of the World Health Assembly.

In the same year Rotary, WHO, UNICEF, and the CDC formed the Global Polio Eradication Initiative. As in the Americas, the greatest challenge within developing countries was the lack of infrastructure, particularly when it came to surveillance; if GPEI wanted all the reports from different countries to add up to a meaningful whole, they had to standardize the procedures and reports. Walt Dowdle, then deputy director of the CDC, recalls: "Managing data, standardizing surveillance, and collecting specimens was an enormous job. There were 148 accredited labs around the world. A first tier of labs did the first examination for the virus, and the upper tier of labs did all of the RNA analysis."[2]

As the core team faced this and other challenges, they were bolstered by the readiness of Rotary to take on roles beyond those typically played by donors. With members spread across 23,000 communities in 161 countries, Rotary was a unique resource in global health. India, for example, experienced about 70 percent of the polio cases reported across the world. With seventy-three Rotary clubs in Mumbai alone, Rotary was an enormous political and volunteer force. Rotary leaders advocated for India to sponsor National Immunization Days (NIDs), and when India decided to do so, Rotary fielded 350,000 volunteers (including members, family, and friends). They turned out to immunize children in booths that had been set up and, in the following two days, went house-to-house to find any child who had not been immunized. Other organizations joined in the effort, including India's National Social Service and the National Cadet Corps. Thanks to such efforts, India's first NID, held in 1995, reached 82 million children.[3]

The other partnering organizations of GPEI also demonstrated real commitment, and the impact of their efforts reflects that commitment and the collaborative spirit behind it. Although the GPEI effort has not yet led to full eradication, its success has resonated throughout the world. According to researchers at the Harvard School of Public Health (reporting in 2007), "in 1988, the year the World Health Assembly resolved to eliminate the poliovirus, polio was endemic in 125 countries, with an estimated 350,000 cases of paralytic polio occurring each year. Today, polio remains endemic in only four countries—Nigeria, Pakistan, Afghanistan, and India— and the total number of reported cases worldwide for the last several years has been less than two thousand."[4] GPEI was so successful in the end, says Dowdle, that "other collaborative areas in infectious diseases now recognize the standards set by polio."[5]

This partnership not only demonstrates the essential role a donor can play in funding and guiding multiple projects over a period of many years; it also provides a glimpse at roles donors can play *outside* the funding arena. In the case of Rotary, the direct involvement of Rotary International chapters in developing key relationships inside targeted countries proved to be a strong asset.

In every successful partnership we profiled, donors played a highly supportive role that extended beyond the usual funding role—providing strategic guidance, supporting local area infrastructure, and encouraging collaboration between partners. "Donors," we realized, played important nonfunding roles, and the combination of those roles with the power of sustained funding represented an extremely important resource for promoting collaboration

Based on the various roles donors played in these partnerships (and based

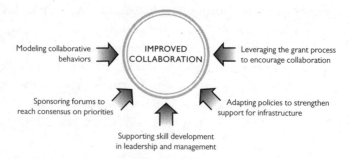

FIGURE 10.1   Ways donors can encourage collaboration. **Donors have opportunities outside traditional funding to encourage real collaboration and improve impact.**

on the needs that came to our attention), we have defined several possibilities outside traditional funding for donors to encourage real collaboration and improve impact (Figure 10.1). The focus of these recommendations is not on dramatic increases in funding but on policies and targeted initiatives that can serve as levers for improving collaboration.

We recognize that donors have been calling for greater collaboration in global health for many years. We also know they face constraints, given their resources and the convictions of their own donors. We offer the ideas in this chapter in the hope that the donor community will use its influence and resources to become a collective catalyst for more effective collaboration, but with the realization that individual donor organizations are not free to act on every recommendation.

LEVERAGE GRANTS TO ENCOURAGE COLLABORATION WITHIN SPECIFIC PARTNERSHIPS

The heart of close collaboration is the partner group itself—the individuals who arrive with different perspectives to try to reach a single goal. Whether they will become a team that can share ideas openly and solve problems together hangs in the balance when they meet for the first time. Donors can help disseminate the lessons for making that happen by adopting grant policies that incorporate appropriate rewards and incentives as well as by holding recipients accountable for effective collaboration practices. Below are our suggestions for donors.

Require explicit statements about how collaboration will occur over the course of the project. For example, donors might require partnerships to respond to such questions as the following:

- How will the partners work with each other?
- How will the partnership provide for feedback from individual partners?
- How will resources be used to support meetings and other means of communication between partners?
- How will the partners work with the ministries of health and finance in the countries being served?

Provide guidance on how the impact of the particular project should be measured. As we described in Chapter 7, global health leaders are only beginning to learn how to measure their progress in terms of impact rather than process. Our advisory group suggested that donors work closely with potential grant recipients to help them design an effective way to evaluate their efforts—for example, providing potential partnerships with examples of how teams have measured progress in similar efforts (drawing from outside as well as inside global health).

Emphasize the critical First Mile activities described earlier, including agreement on membership, goal, structure, strategy, and organizational roles. If partners make decisions about these elements with deliberation, full participation, and understanding, the project is likely to move forward much more readily. If not, the lack of clarity and agreement can lead to delays and frustration. Sally Stansfield, executive secretary of the Health Metrics Network (HMN) and formerly the associate director of global health strategies for the Gates Foundation, recalls one instance: "GAVI

> "I think grantees should come up with how they are willing to be evaluated. They should be willing to say, 'If we don't achieve this, we fail.'"
>
> BILL FOEGE, Senior adviser, Bill & Melinda Gates Foundation, October 19, 2006, interview

has spent a lot of time on damage control and rethinking their governance structure because they ended up with several governance structures that were not well thought out."[6] The importance of early discussions about these foundational elements lies not only in preventing misunderstanding; these discussions also represent a process essential to developing real collaboration. As partnerships make their way through discussions of membership, goal, structure, strategy, and organizational roles, they are building relationships—the critical underpinning that determines the success or failure of their work together.

Donors can encourage thoughtful discussions by building an expectation into grants that several meetings will be required in the First Mile phase of the project and that these meetings should thoroughly explore critical elements until consensus is reached. Individual partner feedback can alert the partnership and donor(s) about any elements that are not clearly understood and agreed upon. In some cases donors might want to encourage potential partners to undertake the work of the First Mile after an initial development grant has been awarded and make subsequent funding contingent on successful completion of the First Mile tasks.[7]

Give grantees resources to use for learning how to develop real collaboration and improve effectiveness of partnerships. For example, donors might develop a cadre of senior fellows from all sectors who are experienced in global health and willing to work on-site with partnerships at critical stages in a project. Donors might also convene retreats for multiple teams that are experiencing similar challenges, with each team presenting its situation and inviting others to participate in problem solving for the project. Such methods of active learning are likely to be highly effective and should be continued over the lifetime of a partnership.

Create a mechanism for flexibility within grants that allows for innovation and risk taking. For example, donors might designate some portion of the grant in unrestricted funds to allow partnerships to take advantage of opportunities as they arise. Otherwise, partnerships may not take risks and push the envelope.

Provide partnerships with reasonable assurance of sustainability so they can confidently plan their activities, particularly their work with local organizations. Developing real collaboration takes time, so donors need to offer assurance of funding for a sustained period (if requirements are met). Currently, partnerships face uncertainties from every funding source.

Although developing countries often provide a portion of funding, that source can present difficulties if the country's budgeting process does not coincide with the timing of a program's activities. And foundations can also be unreliable due to donor fatigue, new leaders or board members, and new benefactors. Bilaterals often demonstrate a similar level of inconsistency. At our symposium for global health leaders, Mike Merson of Yale University, who directed WHO's Global Program on AIDS from 1990 to 1995, cited the "inconsistency and impatience" of bilaterals as one of the major difficulties of partnerships.[8] In general, says Seth Berkley of the International AIDS Vaccine Initative (IAVI), "donor organizations typically don't stick with initiatives. . . . This is very disruptive. The changes in direction make it very hard to have sustained, long-term impact."[9] This uncertainty—not knowing if a project will be sustained—discourages individuals from putting in the hard work required to develop real collaboration.

With all of these issues in mind, donors need to look beyond traditional funding strategies and generate fresh approaches that reward success with sustainability. Partnerships that fail to reach their milestones and other hurdles need to be disbanded. Those that succeed in reaching their milestones and other hurdles need to have assurance funding will continue. Jim Kim suggests that "funders should construct the funding to allow them to evaluate the coalition on an ongoing basis to determine whether all members are pulling their weight and whether they are effective in solving the public health problem."[10] Assurance of sustainability, as part of grant provisions, would provide enormous leverage in encouraging partnerships to become real collaborations. As Bill Foege said in his closing remarks at the symposium, "With foundations and donors, the great power comes at the beginning before you ever give out money. It's the possibility of money that allows you to promote a certain kind of coalition."[11]

"Projects must be sustainable for the recipients, which means integrating them with local health systems and empowering local officials wherever possible. . . . This means that corporations must make a long-term commitment and have the sound financial base to live up to it."

RAYMOND V. GILMARTIN, Former CEO, Merck & Company, Inc., quoted in "A New Role for Corporate America," *Global Health Leadership and Management*

ADAPT POLICIES TO STRENGTHEN SUPPORT FOR INFRASTRUCTURE

One of the unavoidable burdens of partnerships conducting interventions is the lack of infrastructure in developing countries—from the lack of staff to the lack of skills, financial resources, and information systems in public health ministries. In Africa, for example, health-care workers are needed. In Eastern Europe workers are in reasonable supply, but buildings and information systems are inadequate. In many countries the lack of financial skills leads to problems in handling the financial requirements of funders

Ironically, donor efforts to address the issues often have unintended consequences. For example, consultants are a typical solution to these problems, but it's a solution that lacks sustainability. When donors encourage the use of consultants in lieu of helping locals build their own skills, they are contributing to problems for future projects. Donors can also undermine projects by providing the funds to conduct the projects but no money for the infrastructure to manage them.

Donors can ease the burden on developing countries and contribute to infrastructure development by adapting their policies in several ways. Below are five suggestions for policy changes to support infrastructure development.

Standardize grant requirements to minimize the reporting burden on developing countries. Michel Sidibé, deputy executive director of UNAIDS, told participants at the symposium that his team went to 131 countries and asked them to define obstacles to improving health. A common obstacle was the proliferation of partnerships at the country level.[12] "One country had 150 AIDS missions in one year," he said. "They cannot respond to that and still do implementation." For major funders alone, district managers and medical officers spend close to 50 percent of their time writing reports, according to Michael Conway of McKinsey & Company, a panelist who had conducted a study for the Gates Foundation. To lessen the pressure, donors might reduce the number of reports they require and work together to develop standard protocols, approaches to surveillance and evaluation, and approaches to other common grantee requirements.

View each partnership as an opportunity to build local skills. Developing countries do not have the resources to build capabilities and are reliant on donors for such improvements. One of the most important capabilities they need is the capability to integrate the goals and coordinate the programs of different donors. This type of coordination is most likely to succeed when it is managed from within rather than imposed from outside the country. At the symposium Bill Foege said, "I think donors should also be asking, in addition to whatever they are giving the money for, 'How does this improve infrastructure in the long run?'"[13]

One way to support local skills is to provide a line item for overhead costs incurred in implementing grants. A 2005 joint report by the Gates Foundation and McKinsey & Company, *Global Health Partnerships: Assessing Country Consequences*, suggests that donors support such overhead costs.[14] "This will allow countries to build the management capacity and technical infrastructure needed to implement grant activities."[15]

Another avenue is to require partnerships in some countries to involve local professionals in implementing projects. Seth Berkley describes how IAVI has supported infrastructure development in this way: "A lot of money is being spent on clinical trials. The NIH typical structure is to give it to U.S. academic institutions whose incentive is to build their own capacities to get more money. IAVI has a different approach of empowering the scientists, researchers, and partners in the developing country. As a result, they are able to do trials in eleven countries. This has worked remarkably well. In Kenya they are on the fifth trial."[16]

Develop channels for ensuring that "the voice of the South" is heard. For example, donors might develop a method of gathering feedback from program recipients. This feedback can help improve programs in many ways—for example, helping multiple donors understand how to integrate efforts. In addition to gathering feedback, donors might consider supporting the attendance of representatives from developing countries at global health meetings, to assure their perspective is heard and contribute to their skill building.

Consider creative ideas from grantees for incorporating development of health

---

"We tend to overwhelm countries. Collaboration is a huge challenge at the country level. It's more complex than at the global level."

SUSAN HOLCK, Director, general management, WHO, Coalitions and Collaboration in Global Health: A Symposium for Global Health Leaders, October 19–20, 2006

monitoring and evaluation systems into projects. There are no obvious answers to filling the information systems gap under present funding approaches. Even though the health information system of a recipient country might serve as an integrating force for the contributions of various donors, those donors are currently unlikely to fund that system. Alan Hinman, a senior public health scientist at the Task Force for Global Health, says: "What everyone asks is, 'How many lives did we save?' The challenge is to make effective use of the categorical funding to build infrastructure. . . . We need to get people in rich countries committed to a categorical intervention that forces you to build health information systems for chronic, enduring care."[17]

A DFID report published in 2004 also suggests the idea of "donors top slicing their contribution to the financing GHPs (Global Health Partnerships), so that a given percentage is withheld from the overall donation."[18] This funding could be used for monitoring and evaluation systems.

Whatever the mechanism, donors need to find ways to support the development of health information systems in recipient countries so partnerships, donors, and the countries themselves have a better basis for setting priorities and tracking progress.

Support broad efforts for standardizing data collection. Closely related to the need for information systems development within recipient countries is the need to standardize the types of data collected across regions. Sally Stansfield was involved with starting the Health Metrics Network in 2005, while at the Gates Foundation. She describes why standardization is important:

> Through the years, donors have initiated and funded their own priorities in each country and have allocated significant resources to the measurement, monitoring, and evaluation of health status programs. Such support has

---

"In our view, the only long-term sustainable goal for donors and developing countries is to build indigenous capacity for innovation to ensure the effectiveness of health systems."

TARA ACHARYA, Consultant, Rockefeller Foundation
CHARLES A. GARDNER, Head of Innovation Program, Global Forum for Health Research
DEREK YACH, Director, Global Health, Rockefeller Foundation
Technological Innovation, Social Innovation, and the Role of Developing Countries in Global Health

---

often improved data availability and use. However, it has also had some unintended negative effects . . . producing information that cannot be compared between countries over time, that are not trusted by decision makers and not used to improve health-service delivery, leaving the global community with no comparability across countries.[19]

To improve data collection across regions, donors need to join forces to provide technology for regional monitoring of disease efforts and to standardize data collection.

In developing regional standards, donors from various sectors need to bring together the data collectors and data users from the targeted countries and regions to define their joint data requirements. As David Ross of the Public Health Informatics Institute cautions, standardization cannot be accomplished from the top down: "Experience has taught us three important things: First, every community will think their needs are unique and will be skeptical that common needs can be defined. Second, you won't get cooperation if you try to manage the effort top-down. And, third, the people who will ultimately collect and use the data have valuable insights to offer."[20]

By acting on these five suggestions for policy changes to support infrastructure development, donors can improve the impact of their programs while empowering recipient countries to play a stronger role in public health.

SUPPORT DEVELOPMENT OF LEADERSHIP AND MANAGEMENT SKILLS

The third way donors can encourage collaboration is by supporting the development of leadership and management skills among global health participants. Global health is rich in intelligent and experienced leaders from all sectors and geographic areas, North and South, who dedicate their lives to their work. But the complex demands of partnerships require skills that many people have not had the opportunity to develop. Partners who come from the private sector and the social sciences may have access to leadership and management training as part of the natural course of their professional lives, but those from public health and the medical sciences are less likely to encounter such training as part of their undergraduate or postgraduate experiences. They could benefit from project management training that includes budgeting, personnel management, and communication, for instance.[21] They could also benefit from leadership training in such areas as vision, strategy, and team development. In addition, leaders from all sectors could benefit from training that addresses the complexities of dealing with international cultural diversity, infrastructure issues, and other circumstances particular to global health projects.

A number of leaders in global health education suggested that it would be very difficult to teach collaborative leadership skills in the context of MPH programs because most students are young and have not had enough real-world experience in working collaboratively to appreciate the importance of these skills. Instead, they suggested that donors can take an active role in helping to develop these skills in midcareer and senior leaders. Donors can encourage the development of leadership and management skills by providing support for NGOs and institutions that express an interest in the area. For example, donors might endow chairs at universities, fund fellowships at NGOs or successful partnerships, invest in centers of leadership, or fund the development of case materials for leadership and management, based on successful collaborations. As Jim Kim of Harvard Medical School says, "I think we're just beginning to build a science of scale-up in global health. I know more about how Southwest Airlines works—from business school case studies—than how smallpox was eradicated. Smallpox should be one of the cases used to teach the new science of 'global health delivery.'"[22]

Such cases would not only be useful in training; they could also serve as reference points for practitioners. On this point, Michel Sidibé says, "For example, if I were looking at an opportunity to create a coalition for a totally different problem, I would need a vision of what it could look like. I would need to know what works under what conditions and what doesn't work. That would help future initiatives in a concrete way."[23] Donors can contribute not only by funding the development of cases, but also by sharing the lessons learned from successful and unsuccessful programs.

> "Perhaps a traditional way to think about business is 'Write us a big check, please, and then go away.' That's leaving a lot of value on the table. . . . I think what is emerging is that business can bring other competencies to the solution."
>
> JAMES AUSTIN, Professor emeritus, Harvard Business School, Coalitions and Collaboration in Global Health: A Symposium for Global Health Leaders, October 19–20, 2006

Collaborations in global health often fall short because it is difficult to translate the attitude and concept of collaboration into concrete applications. We believe that effective collaboration can be taught, but it requires active learning and ongoing coaching, and it cannot be taught in a single lecture or even through one very-well-written paper or book. Donors are in an excellent position to connect their grantees with the individuals and organizations that can provide skill building in collaboration that goes beyond simply understanding a particular set of principles or guidelines. These resources can provide instruction and guidance as the grantees actually struggle in real time with building, strengthening, and maintaining their coalition. This is the process of active learning. Active learning is based in the philosophy of "learning by doing," where the tools and techniques learned are applied directly to a real-life situation.

Because the resources that could provide this active learning in building partnerships are scarce, the participants at the Carter Center symposium suggested that we establish a Center for Global Health Collaboration that would act as a resource center for making these tools and techniques available to professionals working in global health. This center was subsequently established in 2008 and based at The Task Force for Global Health. Its purpose is to build the necessary skill base for more effective collaboration, provide systematic evidence for how these techniques can make a demonstrable improvement in collaborative outcomes, and serve as a global technical resource to improve the chances that partnerships will be successful.

Donors from the business sector can play a special role by providing faculty for management training at leadership centers or becoming more active in providing consulting services to partnerships, building the skills of public-sector partners along the way. A 2003 special edition of the *McKinsey Quarterly* cited several instances of such services, while noting they were "still distressingly rare."[24]

SPONSOR FORUMS FOR GLOBAL HEALTH LEADERS TO REACH CONSENSUS ON PRIORITIES

In the absence of an overall architecture in global health, donors can also play an important role by sponsoring forums for global health leaders from all sectors to create a consensus on key priorities.

Bring together those leaders who are working on a particular disease or

threat, so they can reach consensus about the best ways to coordinate efforts.
Clearly, donors would have greater impact if they coordinated efforts to
address a particular disease or threat. Yet in his opening remarks at the
symposium, President Jimmy Carter observed, "There's no coordination
that I can detect in the treatment of AIDS. It's a piecemeal approach. We
need to analyze what the needs are and who could provide those needs."[25]
Jim Kim, who formerly directed WHO's HIV/AIDS department, returned
to the topic in a panel discussion on the disease:

> Before I went to WHO, the U.S. government decided it would follow its
> own path on HIV/AIDS. I don't know of any other time with a major disease
> that the United States decided to do that. In the early days there was effec-
> tively a firewall between WHO and PEPFAR [the principal U.S. overseas aid
> program for AIDS, TB, and Malaria]. PEPFAR's insistence on targets and
> monitoring quality have led to some great successes. But in my view, the
> most important achievements in the history of global health were the result
> of truly collaborative efforts involving both individual governments and
> multilateral institutions like WHO. HIV is not a problem that can be solved
> by a single nation.[26]

While HIV/AIDS drew the most comment, symposium participants raised
the same issue for other diseases and health threats and suggested forums
for each major disease and threat to coordinate efforts.[27]

Mike Merson of Yale suggested how a forum on a specific disease/threat
might work: "The best way is to bring together a group of good thinkers for
a retreat for a few days who know the disease and know the UN and bilateral
systems. Let people present where we are and analyze what is needed and
the best way to get there. They need to be a mixture of people—Americans
and non-Americans, developing country leaders and developed country
leaders. It should be doable if we can identify the right people."[28] As the
panelists pointed out, forum participants also need to select a team of
leaders who will implement their decisions, rather than delegating the task
to individuals at lower levels in their organizations who were not involved
in the discussions.

*Hold a series of donor coordination conferences, each focused on a specific
country.* Donors have been taking steps to coordinate activities with other
donors since the 1980s, but the rapid rise in the numbers of donors serving

an individual country indicates a broader effort is needed. Such conferences might begin with presentations by leaders from the recipient country about their needs and difficulties, followed by presentations by donors, citing their own constraints and concerns. The goal would be to agree on ways to improve donor coordination and health impact and to select leaders from each conference to implement the decisions. The summary of such conferences would also provide a useful profile of infrastructure needs for each country that could be broadly communicated across global health.

Convene forums for discussing priorities across global health and how efforts can be coordinated. Michael Conway of McKinsey suggested that "the debate should be an analysis of how well we're doing in addressing global health issues and what should change." In fact, in 2007, the year after the Carter Center symposium, senior global health leaders from eight international organizations met in New York to discover ways to collaborate better.[29] One of their five action items included "development of a framework for mutual accountability that would lead to clear roles and responsibilities and a system for monitoring commitments." Such a system would lay the foundation for the analysis Conway suggests.

Forums to set priorities should also include participants from recipient countries. On this need, Nils Daulaire of the Global Health Council said, "The premise has been: get smart people together and they'll figure it out. But we're dealing with complex adaptive systems. . . . People in the community have to be part of the process."[30] The goal of the forum would be to develop a set of priorities and the roles organizations would take in addressing each.

Some would like to see such debates linked to the UN's Millennium

Development Goals. Paul Zeitz, the executive director of Global AIDS Alliance, commented: "We could come up with a global strategic plan for achieving the MDGs [millennium development goals] by 2015. We have a big goal, but we don't have a plan."[31] If a series of forums could produce agreement about which organizations would assume responsibility for each goal or initiative (with a method of tracking), the basis could be established for such a plan. These ideas for donor-sponsored forums will require that one or more large donors take the initiative and serve as convener, ideally a foundation or an NGO that can play an objective role. According to those global health leaders who provided input for this book, broad support for such a step currently exists.

MODEL COLLABORATIVE BEHAVIORS

Those we interviewed and those who attended the symposium also called on donors to model collaborative behavior, strengthening their capacity to work with their own organizational units as well as external partners. The following five ideas came out of the discussions:

1. *Take only joint credit when funding joint projects, suppressing egos just as highly collaborative leaders do.* As Anu Gupta, a director of contributions for Johnson & Johnson, remarked, "It's hypocritical to tell recipients they need to collaborate if donors are not going to model collaboration. . . . Donors need to turn 'I' into 'we' and give everyone credit."[32]

2. *Create a nonprejudicial method for receiving recipient feedback.* Donors need to be good listeners and have reasonable feedback loops from the recipients; otherwise they will not be in a position to appropriately support these collaborations. Current mechanisms fail to address the issue of grantees' fear of repercussions. Possible mechanisms might include third-party interviews or group forums in which grantees are encouraged to raise issues.

3. *Create a donor watch that monitors donor results.* A number of global health leaders expressed support for the idea of a donor watch. It could start with each donor's stated mission, using such metrics as life expectancy and such methods as household surveys to measure

success against that mission. Anil Soni of the Clinton Foundation pointed out that this practice would "put donors on the hook to be responsible to make coalitions work, rather than saying, 'Here's how things work.'" Armin Fidler of the World Bank added, "If an organization had the capacity and breadth to really evaluate what we're doing and put this information on the Web, it would be an important trigger for more partnerships and collaborations."[33]

4. *Work in tandem within a country.* Donors might adopt a policy of jointly visiting recipient countries whenever possible. As Fidler commented, "When organizations like WHO and the World Bank make joint visits, it's a signal to the country leaders that they're truly working together. Countries notice that."[34]

5. *Create a workshop for staff members.* The workshop should focus on the ingredients for success in real collaboration, so staff members can contribute ideas for improving collaboration in partnerships and serve as role models themselves.

These ideas for modeling collaborative behavior are just a beginning. Donors themselves are in the best position to craft such behaviors, and the forums suggested would provide an excellent way to exhibit them. A quiet demonstration of complementary leadership roles at such forums and joint credit in the printed materials and Web site information would communicate more about collaboration than any number of speeches or articles.

In this chapter we've described many steps donors can take to leverage their special position in global health partnerships. No group of organizations has a similar power to change behaviors. Through their traditional

"Despite having significantly fewer resources than government, the philanthropic sector is needed to play a catalytic role in launching new initiatives, providing early funding, and evaluating in flexible, creative ways the question of how best to use the limited resources in global health."

GORDON CONWAY, Former president, Rockefeller Foundation, "Partnering to Develop New Products for Diseases of Poverty," November 2004

roles as grant makers and their less traditional roles of bringing together leaders across global health and promoting collaborative skills, donors can lead improvements in the success of global health efforts that will benefit countless lives.

NOTES

1. Pandak, interview with the authors, March 17, 2006.
2. Dowdle, interview with the authors, December 21, 2004.
3. Pigman, *Conquering Polio,* 41–63.
4. Nankin, "Prevention: It Just Makes Cents," 1–2.
5. Dowdle, interview with the authors, December 21, 2004.
6. Stansfield, interview with the authors, June 10, 2005.
7. See the "First Mile Toolkit" at the back of this book.
8. Merson's comments are from Coalitions and Collaboration in Global Health: A Symposium for Global Health Leaders, October 19, 2006.
9. Berkley, interview with the authors, January 4, 2005.
10. Kim, interview with the authors, November 16, 2004.
11. These comments are from Foege's closing remarks at Coalitions and Collaboration in Global Health: A Symposium for Global Health Leaders, October 20, 2006.
12. See Sidibé's visual, Figure 2.4, in Chapter 2.
13. Foege's comments are from the Coalitions and Collaboration in Global Health: A Symposium for Global Health Leaders, October 20, 2006.
14. The report, *Global Health Partnerships: Assessing Country Consequences,* is available online at http://www.hlfhealthmdgs.org/Documents/GatesGHPNov2005.pdf.
15. Ibid., 24.
16. Berkley, interview with the authors, January 4, 2005.
17. Hinman, interview with the authors, March 10, 2006.
18. Caines, *Assessing the Impact of Global Health Partnerships,* 5.
19. Stansfield, interview with the authors, June 10, 2005.
20. Ross, interview with the authors, January 6, 2005.
21. Jacob Kumaresan of the International Trachoma Initiative mentioned the need for these three skills at an advisory group meeting with the authors, November 11, 2005.
22. Kim, interview with the authors, March 10, 2006.
23. Sidibé's comments are from Coalitions and Collaboration in Global Health: A Symposium for Global Health Leaders, October 20, 2006.
24. Gupta and Taliento, "How Businesses Can Combat Global Disease," 100–3.
25. Carter's comments are from his opening remarks at Coalitions and Collaboration in Global Health: A Symposium for Global Health Leaders, October 19, 2006.
26. Kim's comments are from Coalitions and Collaboration in Global Health: A Symposium for Global Health Leaders, October 19, 2006.

27. Such forums may also be useful for sharing prospective research on conducting interventions.

28. Merson's comments are from Coalitions and Collaboration in Global Health: A Symposium for Global Health Leaders, October 20, 2006.

29. The meeting took place on July 19, 2007, and included senior leaders from WHO, the Global Fund, GAVI, the UNFPA, the World Bank, UNAIDS, UNICEF, and the Gates Foundation.

30. Daulaire's comments are from Coalitions and Collaboration in Global Health: A Symposium for Global Health Leaders, October 20, 2006.

31. Zeitz's comments are from Coalitions and Collaboration in Global Health: A Symposium for Global Health Leaders, October 20, 2006.

32. Gupta's comments are from Coalitions and Collaboration in Global Health: A Symposium for Global Health Leaders, October 20, 2006.

33. Soni's and Fidler's comments are from Coalitions and Collaboration in Global Health: A Symposium for Global Health Leaders, October 20, 2006.

34. Fidler, in ibid.

Chapter 11 | CONCLUSION
The Purpose of Real Collaboration

Throughout this book we've described an exceptional kind of partnership—the kind that becomes an integrated team and then goes on to achieve far more than anyone anticipated. Like author Jim Collins in his book *Good to Great in the Social Sectors* and Jon Katzenbach and Douglas Smith in *The Wisdom of Teams,* we're talking about excellence and the rewards it brings.[1] We chose this focus because the rewards of dramatically improving human lives are worth the difficulties. We can think of no better way to close this book than to return to the inspiring words of Stephen Lewis, the UN special envoy for HIV/AIDS in Africa. He had recently visited the Beira General Hospital in Mozambique, where this disease, the most destructive of our time, was much in evidence:

> I walk into the women's ward and there are fifty-four beds, but there are eighty to ninety women in the ward. All of them young, all of them in their late teens, twenties, and thirties, almost all of them with AIDS-related illnesses and most of them co-infected by tuberculosis.
> ... and they're lying on the concrete floor of the corridor,
> ... and they're lying on the floor between the beds,
> ... and they're lying on the floor under the beds.
> How is this possible? You know that it's happening because of the failure of the world ... to join together and respond to the pandemic, to defeat it, to collaborate with each other in the service of keeping these women alive.[2]

It is our hope that with real collaboration, the work that global health workers do *will* help to keep these women alive and bring to all of them and their families a real chance for leading healthy, safe, and productive lives.

NOTES

1. Collins, *Good to Great in the Social Sectors*; and Katzenbach and Smith, *Wisdom of Teams*.
2. Lewis, interview with the authors, October 19, 2006.

The First Mile Toolkit

As a participant in a newly launched global health project, you are about to begin the exciting yet sometimes daunting First Mile. As pointed out in Chapter 5, the First Mile of a partnership is characterized by optimism and a sense of possibility, but it can also be intimidating. To make the task a little less overwhelming, we have provided you with a toolkit.

In the following pages are tools that can help the partners accomplish the important tasks of this stage:

- Choose the right membership
- Develop a shared goal
- Select the appropriate structure
- Shape a strategy
- Clarify organizational roles

In addition to these "elements" of the First Mile, two additional tools are provided that deal with ground rules for interaction and topics to include in the charter.

Element	Tools
Membership	Stakeholder analysis for potential member organizations
	Stakeholder analysis for potential individual members
Shared goal	Worksheet for developing goal, vision, and mission statements
Structure	Worksheet for decision-making protocol
Strategy	Strengths, weaknesses, opportunities, and threats (SWOT) analysis
	Opportunity matrix
	Strategy worksheet
	Questions for determining key activities
Roles	Questions to determine organizational roles
	Additional tools
	Ground rules for interaction
	Topics to include in charter

STAKEHOLDER ANALYSIS FOR POTENTIAL MEMBER ORGANIZATIONS

As stated in Chapter 6, once a core team has defined key stakeholder groups, it must consider which groups are needed as members and which should participate in such forums as conferences, advisory teams, or community gatherings. It may be necessary to gain a thorough understanding of each organization before deciding how it could positively contribute to the collaboration. This can be accomplished through an analysis of each organization's agenda, potential contributions (human, financial, or technical resources), potential constraints, and possible problems it may present as a member organization.

Organization	Organizational agenda	What can they contribute?	What are their constraints?	What problems can we anticipate?

1. *Organizations.* As a group, identify every organization that will affect or be affected by your initiative. List these organizations in the first column.

2. *Organizational agenda.* Ask volunteers to research each organization's vision and mission as well as its current projects. How well do the organization's activities and goals coincide with those of the partnership?

3. *Contributions.* As a group, discuss the next three columns, starting with contributions. What can the organization contribute? This could entail many things, such as financial or staff resources, field workers, political influence, and so on. When completing this column, it is also helpful to specify what phase of the project is relevant to each stakeholder and their potential contributions.

4. *Constraints.* In what ways is this organization constrained? Constraints could be legal, economic, political, technical, or geographic in nature, to name a few possibilities. Also, are there any partner constraints? For example, conflicts of interest may prevent some organizations from working together.

5. *Problems to anticipate.* By identifying problems that could arise while working with each organization, the core team can consider possible solutions in advance, in order to avoid a time- and resource-consuming clash of opinions. For example, is the organization known for a style of management that could cause problems in the partnership.

STAKEHOLDER ANALYSIS FOR POTENTIAL INDIVIDUAL MEMBERS

This analysis of potential individual members can be accomplished through a discussion of various personal characteristics: influence and authority, experience and skills, personal agenda, and indicators of teamwork.

Stakeholder	Influence and authority	Experience and skills (technical, problem-solving)	Personal agenda/reasons for joining the team	Indicators of teamwork/ positive outlook

1. *Stakeholders.* Get the group together to brainstorm and identify every potential member, and list them in the first column.

2. *Influence and authority.* What connections does this person have (within his or her organization) to high-level leadership and/or to external stakeholders who are important to the project's success? How much influence does the person have in different populations/groups that will be instrumental in project development and implementation?

3. *Experience and skills.* What past projects and initiatives has this person been involved with? What skills did he or she demonstrate in these programs (for example, technical, problem-solving, networking, and so on)?

4. *Personal agenda.* Why would this person want to join the team? If the person comes from a large organization, why is he or she the best representative for this partnership, as opposed to someone else from the same organization?

5. *Indicators of teamwork.* Does this person have experience in working with teams? If so, were those initiatives successful?

WORKSHEET FOR DEVELOPING GOAL, VISION, AND MISSION STATEMENTS

When starting a partnership, with many different agendas coming together, reaching consensus can be difficult. Agreeing on a clear goal, vision, and mission in the beginning helps lay the foundation for consensus on other issues. Developing the goal, vision, and mission statements should be an exercise in *real collaboration*, with all member organizations represented in the discussion. The following worksheet contains spaces that can be filled in during the process of developing the partnership goal, vision, and mission statements. The notes that follow this table give suggestions for how, when, and by whom each space can be filled in.

	Goal	*Vision*	*Mission*
Definitions	What is the partnership's target outcome? The goal should be focused and clear, addressing *affected populations*, *timeframe*, and *measurements of success,* and members need to have a shared understanding of its meaning.	What change will be seen in the world if the partnership achieves the goal?	What is the purpose of the partnership?
Premeeting Planning	Facilitator: Timetable: Examples: Discussion questions:	Facilitator: Timetable: Examples: Discussion questions:	Facilitator: Timetable: Examples: Discussion questions:

	Goal	Vision	Mission
Group discussion	Brainstorm elements:	Brainstorm elements:	Brainstorm elements:
	Agree on key elements:	Agree on key elements:	Agree on key elements:
	Draft possible statements:	Possible statements:	Possible statements:
Fine-tuning	First draft:	First draft:	First draft:
	Partner comments:	Partner comments:	Partner comments:
	Second draft:	Second draft:	Second draft:
	Partner comments:	Partner comments:	Partner comments:
Final statements	Final:	Final:	Final:

1. *Definitions.* The convener or another partner(s) with good facilitation skills needs to prepare for the meeting in advance. To help your team get started, circulate the definitions of goal, vision, and mission to all partners and encourage them to think about what they want the partnership's goal, vision, and mission to be.
2. *Premeeting planning.* Before the partners meet, the convener may also want to prepare the following:

- *Timetable.* The convener should determine a reasonable time-table for the process. Time should also be allowed for partners to provide feedback before the group discussion takes place. Once that discussion takes place and all group members contribute their opinions, drafts will have to be written by the convener/core group and circulated to the other partners for comments.
- *Examples.* The convener should gather examples of statements from other partnerships to demonstrate the differences between goal, vision, and mission. These example statements can ignite a lively discussion between the partners as they decide what elements they do or do not want to incorporate in their own statements.
- *Discussion questions.* The convener/core group should generate a set of discussion questions to move the process along. These questions should focus on the importance of collaboration and why these partners have decided to join together. For example, to launch a discussion of the goal, the convener might ask, "How will working together help us achieve a goal we cannot meet alone?"

3. *Group discussion.* The group discussion should involve all partners, and the end result should be a list of key elements to be included in the goal, vision, and mission statements. If the partnership is large, small groups for discussion can assure that every partner partici-pates. The following steps may be helpful:
   - *Brainstorm elements.* Using the example statements and discus-sion questions, partners can brainstorm the elements to include in the partnership's goal, vision, and mission. It is important at this stage to show respect for all suggestions.
   - *Agree on key elements.* For this step, partners can go through all of the elements listed during the brainstorming session and decide which of them are truly vital to the partnership. This step will likely provoke differences of opinion, but working through these differences can lead to a greater sense of understanding and trust among the partners.
   - *Possible statements.* The partners can then draft their ideas of what the partnership's goal, vision, and mission should be.

Depending on the number of partners, these possible statements can be drafted by each small group or each individual. The convener should emphasize that "perfect" wording is not the main concern in this step; each small group or individual partner should focus on including all key elements in a coherent statement. These possibilities can then be reported to the larger group to find synergies, eliminate duplication, and allow for the larger group's reaction to the different possibilities.

4. *Fine-tuning.* After the group discussion has taken place, the convener/core group should consider every possible statement that was turned in by the partners. Based on the key elements included in these statements, the convener/core group should draft statements and gather feedback from the partners until a consensus is reached. This stage of the process can include several drafts. It may be helpful for the convener to keep track of the drafts through these steps:

   · *Draft.* Write the drafts into the worksheet to document the evolution of the partnership's goal, vision, and mission.

   · *Partner comments.* Include the feedback received from every partner in these spaces. This will help to produce the next draft. (If several drafts are needed, the worksheet can be expanded.)

5. *Final statements.* At this point consensus should be growing among the partners about the goal, vision, and mission statements. Circulate the final statements to the partners and congratulate yourself and your team for successfully completing this essential task.

WORKSHEET FOR DECISION-MAKING PROTOCOL

In Chapter 6 we described several key elements to laying the foundation for close collaboration: membership, shared goal, structure, strategy, and organizational roles. Once these key elements are established, some partnerships find it helpful to develop a decision-making protocol that defines the level of authority needed to make different types of decisions. This worksheet can be useful for guiding a discussion of this protocol. For each type of decision that may arise in the workings of the partnership, agree on what level of consensus must be reached to make that decision.

	Full partnership	Majority of partnership	Single partner to whom most relevant (specify)	Delegate to (specify)	Broad stakeholder input
Type of decision	☐	☐			☐
New members	☐	☐			☐
Officers	☐	☐			☐
Procedural rules	☐	☐			☐
Budget approval	☐	☐			☐
Expenditures	☐	☐			☐
Charter approval	☐	☐			☐
Policy development	☐	☐			☐
Advocacy statements	☐	☐			☐

SWOT ANALYSIS

Completing an analysis of strengths, weaknesses, opportunities, and threats (SWOT) is an important step in optimizing the strengths and minimizing the weaknesses of your partnership. Work through the SWOT analysis to spark discussions of possibilities the partnership should consider (refer to the elements of the "Stakeholder Analysis for Potential Individual Members" completed earlier to help identify strengths, weaknesses, opportunities, and threats).

EXAMPLE OF SWOT ANALYSIS

	Helpful	*Harmful*
Internal	*Strengths* A strong research component of the partnership allows for flexibility in a changing environment. Solid relationships with political figures in the country will help the partnership's efforts to gain political support.	*Weaknesses* The partnership's funding sources are ever-changing and precarious. The partnership lacks adequate technical support.
External	*Opportunities* The issues the partnership seeks to resolve have been stated as a priority for a potential funder. The country's government has committed to greatly increase health-sector funding.	*Threats* The political landscape seems to be on the verge of transition. Citizens of the country are suspicious of health workers from outside countries.

Strengths. What are the attributes of your partnership that will help to achieve your mission? Think in terms of resource availability, established relationships/contacts, donation capabilities, and so on.

Weaknesses. What are the attributes of your partnership that could hurt your chances of achieving your mission? Focus on the partnership's attributes that might lead to failures and losses or hinder the partnership's adaptive capabilities.

Opportunities. What are some *external* conditions that will help your partnership to achieve its mission? Look at the local, regional, and global environment to brainstorm opportunities. Have any recent changes occurred in technology, government, policy, and so on, that present opportunities to advance your initiatives?

Threats. What are some *external* conditions that could keep your partnership from achieving its mission? For threats, again consider the local, regional, and global landscape to identify potential threats. For example, is there a competing cause, a similar initiative that has received little support in the past, or political instability?

OPPORTUNITY MATRIX

One result of the "SWOT Analysis" is a list of opportunities. The "Opportunity Matrix" provides a format for prioritizing these opportunities, based on two considerations: value and cost/degree of difficulty. Opportunities that fall within the lower end of the "Cost/degree of difficulty" spectrum as well as the higher end of the "Value" spectrum are generally more desirable opportunities to pursue. Conversely, opportunities that fall within the higher end of the "Cost/degree of difficulty" spectrum as well as the lower end of the "Value" spectrum are less desirable opportunities to pursue.

Value. What is the relative importance of the activity to the partnership's mission?

Cost/degree of difficulty. Is this activity particularly costly or difficult to sustain?

	Cost/degree of difficulty	
	Low	*High*
Value *High*	These are going to be your *most* appealing opportunities.	Are these opportunities worth their associated *costs*?
Value *Low*	Are these opportunities *valuable* enough to pursue?	These are going to be your *least* appealing opportunities.

STRATEGY WORKSHEET

Once the significant strengths, weaknesses, threats, and opportunities are identified, it is possible to establish a strategy statement for how the collaboration will go about accomplishing its shared goal. The overall strategy does not need to include the details of specific activities; instead, it should lay out the overall approach. *While developing this strategy, it is important to keep in mind how the collaboration can capitalize on its greatest opportunities and manage its potential threats.*

Goal	Strategy for reaching the goal	Major milestones

This exercise may lead to a one-sentence statement of strategy or two or three strategic initiatives. By discussing these topics, the group can move from the big-picture context to key activities for carrying out the stategy (or strategies) and resources.

QUESTIONS FOR DETERMINING KEY ACTIVITIES

Once the overall strategy for the collaboration is clearly defined, it is possible to break down the strategy into specific activities. When identifying specific activities, four important elements should be considered:

1. What will the timeframe be for this activity (activities should include funding activities)?
2. Who will hold the responsibility for this activity (for example, how can individuals leverage their personal strengths)?
3. What resources and support will be necessary for this activity to be carried out?
4. How will the progress of this activity be measured?

Key activity	Timeframe	Person/ organization responsible	Resources/ support needed	Measurement of progress

QUESTIONS FOR DETERMINING ORGANIZATIONAL ROLES

Before the First Mile is completed, each partner should have a good idea of what his or her organization is going to *contribute* to the partnership, as well as how the partnership will *benefit*. This tool encourages partners to clarify that commitment. Once this worksheet is filled out by a representative of each member organization, a list can be compiled and distributed to the entire partnership to avoid confusion in the future. If any partners disagree with the roles described, the partners can hold a group discussion, using this worksheet as a guide for discussion.

My organization's role	How my organization will benefit	How the partnership will benefit and advance toward the goal

1. *My organization's role.* What will my organization's primary role be within the partnership (for example, fundraising, technical support, policy advice, and so on)?

2. *How my organization will benefit.* How will my organization benefit by carrying out this role within the partnership (for example, the goals of the partnership mirror the goals of my organization, allow my organization to make in-country political contacts, and so on)?

3. *How the partnership will benefit.* How will the partnership benefit if my organization carries out this role (increased resources, increased technical capabilities, media attention, and so on)?

GROUND RULES FOR INTERACTION

Area	*Examples of specific ground rules*
Basic courtesies	Members will turn off cell phones during meetings.
	When a person enters a meeting, the convener will briefly summarize the points covered.
Problem solving and decision making	Members will brainstorm ideas before debate begins.
	The convener will summarize when a consensus appears to have been reached.
Frequency/method of internal communication	The convener will set up biweekly conference calls and quarterly face-to-face meetings.
Frequency/method of external communication	Monthly forums will be set up with the external stakeholders.
Accountability	At the end of meetings the convener will summarize action steps, the persons responsible for each action, and the timing for his or her reports on progress.
Conflict resolution	The convener or other designated member will work directly with those involved in conflict within twenty-four hours of its emergence to help resolve the issues.
The convener's role in meetings	The convener will develop an agenda two weeks before a meeting and circulate it for input.
	During meetings the convener will encourage participation by every partner.

Partnerships bring together a diverse group of stakeholders with different perspectives and experiences. By agreeing on ground rules for interaction at the first meeting, the group can begin to establish an open environment, set the stage for meaningful discussion, and help lay the groundwork for resolving conflicts. This process of developing ground rules can help members set a pattern of respect and cooperation. The format below can be used to guide a discussion and develop a list of agreed-upon ground rules:

Basic courtesies

Problem solving and decision making

Frequency/method of internal
communication

Frequency/method of external
communication

Accountability

Conflict resolution

The convener's role in meetings

Depending on the size of the group and the level of discussion, this exercise will take thirty minutes or more. The following steps will help the convener to guide the discussion.

1. Introduce the exercise by giving examples of ground rules and describing how they will help the partners work together productively.

2. To speed the process and encourage participation, consider agreeing up front that when someone suggests a ground rule, it will be accepted unless opposition is expressed. In other words, silence on the part of the group means "we agree," and the item becomes one of the ground rules.

3. Ask for suggested ground rules and record each on a flip chart. (The worksheet here is a guide for the issues that need to be addressed in developing the ground rules.)

4. Once the group agrees to a set of ground rules it can support and live by, post the ground rules on the wall.

5. Explain that any of the participants can bring attention to how the group is straying from the agreed-upon rules.

TOPICS TO INCLUDE IN THE CHARTER

Developing a formal charter is a useful step for any partnership because it clarifies the critical elements of the partnership's work. The worksheet below can be filled out by the convener following discussions of the earlier tools in this "First Mile Toolkit." After drafting the partnership's charter, the convener will need to circulate it, hold a group discussion, and refine it until all partners are committed to it.

Project mission and milestones

Rationale for project:

Goal and timeframe:

Projected outcome, deliverables, and cost:

Key activities:

Measurements/milestones:

Constraints/limits:

Governance and decision path

Decision path/responsibility for decision making and management:

Timing of key decisions:

Responsibilities of core member organizations

Core member organization:	Resources committed:	Timeframe:

Sponsor/funding commitments

Sponsor:	Resources committed:	Timeframe:

Stakeholders

Key stakeholders:	Stakeholder concerns:

Target recipients/clients:	Needs of recipients/clients:

Strategy for communicating with stakeholders:

SUPPLEMENTARY READING FOR FIRST MILE TOOLS

General

Ancona, D., and D. Caldwell. "Bridging the Boundary: External Activity and Performance in Organizational Teams." *Administrative Science Quarterly* 37 (2001): 634–65.

Aubert, B., and B. Kelsey. "Further Understanding of Trust and Performance in Virtual Teams." *Small Group Research* 34, no. 5 (2003): 575–618.

Barki, H., and A. Pinsonneault. "A Model of Organizational Integration, Implementation Effort, and Performance." *Organization Science* 16, no. 2 (2005): 165–79.

Chinowsky, P., and E. Rojas. "Virtual Teams: Guide to Successful Implementation." *Journal of Management in Engineering* 19, no. 3 (2003): 98.

Duncker, E. "Symbolic Communication in Multidisciplinary Cooperations." *Science, Technology, and Human Values* 26, no. 3 (2001): 349–86.

Jarvenpaa, S., T. Shaw, and D. Staples. "Toward Contextualized Theories of

Trust: The Role of Trust in Global Virtual Teams." *Information Systems Research* 15, no. 3 (2004): 250–67.

Jassawalla, A., and H. Sashittal. "Building Collaborative Cross-Functional New Product Teams." *Academy of Management Executive* 13, no. 3 (1999).

Lasker, R., E. Weiss, and R. Miller. "Partnership Synergy: A Practical Framework for Studying and Strengthening the Collaborative Advantage." *The Milbank Quarterly* 79, no. 2 (2001): 179–205.

Lloyd, J. "Work and Play Well with Others." *Receivables Report for America's Health Care Financial Managers* 19, no. 11 (2004): 6–8.

Marmer, C. "Global Teams—The Ultimate Collaboration." *Personnel Journal* 74, no. 9 (1995).

Weiss, E., R. Anderson, and R. Lasker. "Making the Most of Collaborations: Exploring the Relationship between Partnership Synergy and Partnership Functioning." *Health Education & Behavior* 29, no. 6 (2002): 683–98.

Stakeholders Analysis

Dyer, J., P. Kale, and H. Singh. "When to Ally and When to Acquire." *Harvard Business Review* 82, nos. 7–8 (2004): 108–15.

Hamel, G., Y. Doz, and C. Prahalad. "Collaborate with Your Competitors and Win." Harvard Business Review 67, no. 1 (1989): 133.

The Journey: Management Toolkit

The Journey of a global health partnership will present many challenges—logistical, technical, financial, personal, or social in nature. Chapter 7 includes examples of partnerships that have faced such challenges and emerged even stronger than before. One of the central lessons learned from their experiences is that global health teams need to apply greater management discipline to their efforts. This "Journey: Management Toolkit" provides tools to do so and addresses the following:

Research and planning. Partnerships must apply discipline in research and planning to combat the unexpected but inevitable twists and turns in the journey using a flexible approach. Effective management addresses both short- and long-term goals; these are not stagnant but constantly evolving and must be monitored throughout the partnership's journey. Long-term objectives must be modified in light of short-term progress and vice versa.

Measuring and communicating progress. The second component of the Journey: Management Toolkit focuses on the importance of measuring appropriate targets to monitor the partnership's progress and then communicating this progress to key stakeholders to secure their continued support.

Engaging partners in problem solving. The final process in this toolkit deals with maximizing the effectiveness of partner engagement with a focus on productive meetings and the importance of feedback.

The secretariat or the partner responsible for management will probably take the lead in putting these tools to use, but all members of the core team should be involved in applying them to the partnership's work.

Process	Tools
Researching and planning	Problem statement worksheet
	Opportunity matrix
	Consolidated project plan template
Measuring and communicating progress	Balanced scorecard
	Communications plan template
	Worksheet for sharing credit
Engaging partners in problem solving	Checklist for holding productive meetings
	Partner feedback survey: The 10,000-mile checkup
	Milestone-guided activity debriefing

PROBLEM STATEMENT WORKSHEET

During the Journey, partners must answer many questions that have arisen during the First Mile stage of the project. For example, a team conducting an intervention might research the best way to distribute medications. This research could be used to tailor efforts for a geographic region or population or to address problems that arise unexpectedly. This "Problem Statement Worksheet" provides a way for partners to think through a research effort by considering the six essential factors described below it. (Teams can also use the "Problem Statement Worksheet" to apply discipline in discussing uncertainties and to evaluate individual strategies under consideration.)

CENTRAL QUESTION: What is the issue to be resolved?

Context: Key influencers:

Resource constraints: Criteria for success:

Areas outside the scope of the project:

Approach for finding the answer:

---

1. *Context.* What situation led the team to this question/problem?
2. *Key influencers.* Who will influence the decision on moving forward once the answer to the problem is clear? What other political, economic, and social factors can influence the research effort or initiative?
3. *Resource constraints.* What constraints do you face in conducting the research or solving the problem (such as costs, staff, and timeframe)?
4. *Criteria for success.* What criteria will the partners and other stakeholders use for judging the results of your research or the value of your solution?
5. *Areas outside the scope of the project.* What scope limitations do you recognize—for example, are there geographic areas, target populations, or drugs that you will not include in the research?
6. *Approach for finding the answer.* Evaluate planned research or individual strategies under consideration against these criteria.

OPPORTUNITY MATRIX

A global health partnership will likely have an emergent quality; because of this, the value or cost of certain opportunities may fluctuate or new opportunities may present themselves. Therefore, the "Opportunity Matrix" from the "First Mile Toolkit" is repeated to allow modification during the Journey phase. It provides a format for weighing two considerations for various opportunities: value and cost/degree of difficulty. Use this tool by mapping your opportunities in the appropriate quadrants. Opportunities that fall within the lower end of the "Cost/degree of difficulty" spectrum as well as the higher end of the "Value" spectrum are generally more desirable opportunities to pursue. Conversely, opportunities that fall within the higher end of the "Cost/degree of difficulty" spectrum as well as the lower end of the "Value" spectrum are less desirable opportunities to pursue.

Value. What is the relative importance of the activity to the partnership's mission?

Cost/degree of difficulty. Is this activity particularly costly or difficult to sustain?

		Cost/degree of difficulty	
		Low	*High*
Value	*High*	These are going to be your *most* appealing opportunities.	Are these opportunities worth their associated *costs*?
	Low	Are these opportunities *valuable* enough to pursue?	These are going to be your *least* appealing opportunities.

CONSOLIDATED PROJECT PLAN TEMPLATE

Once the overall strategy and the supporting strategies are established, the next step is developing a project plan. The projects that close collaborations undertake can be very complex, with a variety of activities being conducted by different partners simultaneously. The "Consolidated Project Plan Template" provides a way for teams to clarify when activities will be taking place and who will be responsible for each activity.

Month (Specify the month(s) in which each activity will take place)

Activity name	Start	Finish	Duration	1	2	3	4	5	6	7	8	9	10	11	12	13	14	Responsibility
Activity 1	Month	Month	___	☐	☐	☐	☐	☐	☐	☐	☐	☐	☐	☐	☐	☐	☐	Name 1
Activity 2	Month	Month	___	☐	☐	☐	☐	☐	☐	☐	☐	☐	☐	☐	☐	☐	☐	Name 2
Activity 3	Month	Month	___	☐	☐	☐	☐	☐	☐	☐	☐	☐	☐	☐	☐	☐	☐	Name 3
Activity 4	Month	Month	___	☐	☐	☐	☐	☐	☐	☐	☐	☐	☐	☐	☐	☐	☐	Name 4
Activity 5	Month	Month	___	☐	☐	☐	☐	☐	☐	☐	☐	☐	☐	☐	☐	☐	☐	Name 5

BALANCED SCORECARD

The success of a global health project is determined not only by the impact on targeted populations but also along dimensions such as donor satisfaction, each partner's view of team effectiveness, and program efficiency. A "Balanced Scorecard" can be used to establish measurement standards and performance indicators for each such dimension of project success. This tool gives partners a balanced view of performance that goes beyond traditional financial metrics. Each criterion should have its own measurements of success and performance outcomes. Team members should determine together the measurements they will use to evaluate the activities for each dimension. These metrics should be SMART (Specific, Measurable, Achievable, Realistic, and Timely). The following table indicates what areas may be looked at for improvement. These areas are not exhaustive and are often partnership-specific.

Dimensions (Area of focus)	Types of things to think about
Program impact	Ultimate impact we want to achieve (i.e., number of lives improved or saved)
	Different activities we need to perform and complete (i.e., number of people served in target population, number of drugs distributed, etc.)
	Degree to which we completed each activity in the project plan
Team effectiveness	Number of conflicts that go unresolved
	Number of resources actually provided as compared to those agreed upon
	Percentage of activities completed in the project plan

Program efficiency	Degree to which we met scheduled milestones
	Degree to which we kept expenses within original budget
	Degree to which the budget is followed
Donor satisfaction (How well are we meeting our donor's expectations?)	Timeliness and usefulness of reports
	Adequacy of communication between partners and donors
	Alignment of donor and program values with strategies
	Ability of partners to leverage donor investments / contributions
	Program sustainability and long-term impact

COMMUNICATIONS PLAN TEMPLATE

The process of keeping all the key stakeholders of a global health effort appropriately informed can be difficult because there are typically many different types of stakeholder groups and the best method of reaching each group is distinct. This "Communications Plan Template" provides a way to think through each aspect of delivering appropriate and timely communications to a key stakeholder group.

1. *Audience.* How would you characterize your audience (for example, a funder or a local advocacy group)?
2. *Objective.* What is the purpose of communicating with this audience (for example, to give updates, to get input, or to get approval)?
3. *Message.* What is the underlying message of your partnership's communication with this audience?
4. *Type of communication.* What channel of communication will you use (for example, an e-newsletter, e-mail, or conference call)?

EXAMPLE FOR ONE STAKEHOLDER GROUP

Audience	Objective	Message	Type of communication	Frequency	Responsibility	Feedback method
Primary funder	Give updates on the partnership's progress.	The partnership is on track to achieve our goal.	E-newsletter	Quarterly	Secretariat	Follow-up phone call by a partner

5. *Frequency.* How often should the partnership communicate with this audience (for example, biweekly, monthly, or quarterly)?

6. *Responsibility.* Who is responsible for this type of correspondence (for example, the staff of the secretariat or a partner)?

7. *Feedback method.* How will you learn about the audience's response to the communication?

WORKSHEET FOR SHARING CREDIT

To support the continued success of a project, it's important to be intentional about sharing credit. A partner organization's sustained support often depends on the amount of credit they receive. So the partners may want to discuss what kind of recognition each of their organizations needs.

External stakeholders, such as local officials and local donors, may also need recognition. Adequately sharing credit can help regional or local stakeholders and officials develop a sense of ownership for the program and feel invested enough to sustain it.

The "Worksheet for Sharing Credit" can serve as a guide for partner discussion and a tool for planning. Sharing credit is an important exercise in strengthening any partnership and should be taken seriously. Credit is infinitely divisible. In completing this worksheet, every partner's needs as well as ideas for how to fulfill those needs to ensure their continued involvement in the partnership are acknowledged.

Partnering Organization	Recognition needs	Opportunities for giving credit	Specific activities to give credit

1. *Recognition needs.* Each partner should have the opportunity to speak candidly about how much and what kind of credit its organization will need to continue its support for the partnership. For example, credit could take the form of local media attention, success visible to a governing body, or recognition for acting as the head of the partnership.

2. *Opportunities for giving credit.* This column can be used by the partners to identify outlets and opportunities to provide that credit.

3. *Specific activities to give credit.* Partners can brainstorm specific activities that provide each partnering organization with the appropriate form of credit. (More than one activity can apply to the same opportunity in the previous column.)

CHECKLIST FOR HOLDING PRODUCTIVE MEETINGS

Item	Yes	No	Comments
BEFORE A MEETING			
Does the meeting have a clear objective?	☐	☐	
Has an agenda been created and circulated in advance?	☐	☐	
Did all partners have an opportunity to provide input into creating an agenda?	☐	☐	
Has a meeting place been found, reserved, and confirmed?	☐	☐	
Do meeting ground rules exist?	☐	☐	
Are all partners familiar with these ground rules?	☐	☐	
Is the decision-making process defined and understood by all partners?	☐	☐	
Has someone been designated as the official note taker?	☐	☐	

Item	Yes	No	Comments
Are all partners aware of their particular roles and responsibilities for the meeting?	☐	☐	
Are different partners facilitating different meeting topics?	☐	☐	
Is there an established method of recording unresolved issues for follow-up?	☐	☐	
Has background information on topics to be discussed been sent out in advance?	☐	☐	

AFTER THE MEETING

Item	Yes	No	Comments
Did the facilitator(s) take time at the beginning of the meeting to remind participants of why the issue(s) arose?	☐	☐	
Did the attendees use the ground rules too while participating in the discussion?	☐	☐	
Did the facilitator(s) state consensus as it developed?	☐	☐	
Did everyone participate? If no, what could have been done to achieve full participation?	☐	☐	
Was the discussion of certain issues hindered because critical members were not present?	☐	☐	
Did participants agree on next steps, including issues that remained unresolved by the end of the meeting?	☐	☐	
Were notes taken and distributed in a timely fashion, identifying group decisions, timeline, next steps, and responsibility?	☐	☐	
Did the meeting begin on time and end on time?	☐	☐	

PARTNER FEEDBACK SURVEY: THE 10,000-MILE CHECKUP

This worksheet can be used to gather feedback from individuals before a "10,000-Mile Checkup" discussion involving all members of the partnership. The results of the survey can direct and focus the discussion on the perceived strengths and weaknesses of the partnership. Once again, the members of the partnership should agree on the frequency of this feedback loop, by deciding how often the partner feedback survey will be administered and discussed.

	Poorly	*Well*	*Very well*
How well are we communicating with each other?	❑	❑	❑
How well do we identify and handle conflict?	❑	❑	❑
How well do we capture agreements made in the meetings and monitor progress?	❑	❑	❑
How well do partners communicate decisions following a meeting?	❑	❑	❑
How well is the partnership giving and sharing credit?	❑	❑	❑
How well are we adapting to changes in our environment?	❑	❑	❑
How well are we moving toward our goal?	❑	❑	❑
How well are we operating within our budget?	❑	❑	❑
How well are we meeting our milestones?	❑	❑	❑
How well are partners filling the gaps in leadership that arise?	❑	❑	❑

MILESTONE-GUIDED ACTIVITY DEBRIEFING

When your partnership reaches major milestones, it is helpful to capture lessons learned in a constructive way. Both successes and failures present valuable learning opportunities. When debriefing failures, in particular, it's important to follow four important steps:

1. Admit to making the mistake.
2. Learn from the mistake.
3. Warn others before they make the same mistake.
4. Get over the mistake and move on.

This "Milestone-guided Activity Debriefing" worksheet provides a way to debrief projects and adjust the strategic approach depending on what is or is not working.

Aspect	Notes
Project to be debriefed	
Project time period	
Date and time of debriefing	
Team members and their roles	
Goals/objectives of the project	
What went well?	
What did not go well?	
What did we learn?	
What would we do differently?	
Did we meet our goals? Why or why not? What changes (if any) are needed in our strategy?	
What message would be valuable to spread to others as a warning?	
What actions need to be taken in order for us to accept the mistakes and move on?	

SUPPLEMENTARY READING FOR MANAGEMENT TOOLS

General

Ertel, D. "Alliance Management: a Blueprint for Success." *Financial Executive* 17, no. 9 (2001): 36.

Goodall, K., and J. Roberts. "Repairing Managerial Knowledge Ability over Distance." *Organization Studies* 24, no. 7 (2003): 1153–75.

Mealiea, L., and R. Baltazar. "A Strategic Guide for Building Effective Teams." *Public Personnel Management* 34, no. 2 (2005).

Mitchell, T. "Team Building 101: A Managerial's Guide to Building a Cohesive Team." *Healthcare Registration* (2004): 3–5.

Parnell, J. "Improving the Fit Between Organizations and Employees." *SAM Advanced Management Journal* 63, no. 1 (1998): 35.

Problem Statement Worksheet

Atlanta Communications Group, LLC. *An Introduction to Problem Structuring.* Atlanta: Atlanta Communications Group, 2001.

Communications Plan

Panteli, N., and R. Davison. "The Role of Subgroups in the Communication Patterns of Global Virtual Teams." *IEEE Transactions on Professional Communication* 48, no. 2 (2005).

Holding Meetings

Brown, J., and D. Isaacs. "Conversation as Core Business Process." *The Systems Thinker* 7, no. 10 (1996–97).

The Journey: Leadership Toolkit

As mentioned in Chapter 8, fulfillment of several leadership roles is extremely important in global health partnerships. The most successful partnerships fill the needed leadership roles not through a single, strong individual but through complementary leadership in both internal (team) roles and external roles. Over the life of a partnership, roles assume lesser and greater importance, and one role may actually be played by several people as needed. These tools help partnerships clarify the responsibilities for each of these roles, so the person(s) assuming the role can develop an action agenda.

LEADERSHIP: The Main Menu

Internal team leadership role	Tool
Convener	Assuring effective meeting management
Visionary	Maintaining focus on achieving the overall goal
Strategist	Updating strategy
Team builder	Developing an open partnership culture
	Managing conflict

External leadership role	Tools
Advocate	Getting stakeholders on board
Political influencer	Getting officials on board
Networker	Making and leveraging connections

Overall leadership	Tools
Leadership evaluation	Leadership checkup

WORKSHEET FOR THE CONVENER: ASSURING EFFECTIVE MEETING MANAGEMENT

Whether a partnership is formally chartered or remains informal, someone needs to play the role of the convener. Ideally, this person not only sets up meetings but also facilitates them in a participative manner, setting a tone of open dialogue to create the psychic space that allows members to work together successfully. The person who serves as the convener can use this worksheet as the basis for effectively planning and carrying out meetings. In addition, the convener should make sure that every partner participates in meetings and has the opportunity to communicate ideas on how the partnership should operate.

Participant roles	*Who will fill the role*
Initiating meetings (sending out notices, determining agenda)	
Setting up meetings (choosing location, providing refreshment, etc.)	
Facilitating meetings	
Gatekeeping (making sure all partners participate)	
Surfacing conflicts and problems	
Recording and distributing notes	
Communicating information	
Managing logistics (setting up a phone, P.O. box, and/or use of someone's office and staff)	
Identifying follow-up actions and monitoring progress	
Acknowledging contributions to meeting and progress	

WORKSHEET FOR THE VISIONARY:
MAINTAINING FOCUS ON ACHIEVING THE OVERALL GOAL

One person on the team needs to paint a vision that inspires the partners and helps them maintain their focus on achieving the goal. For this reason the visionary is also the "goal-keeper." This role must be played by someone with a real passion for the issue and the ability to communicate that passion. The visionary in the group can use this worksheet independently, at regular intervals, to personally monitor how well the partners are maintaining their focus on the goal or to reflect on how well he or she is providing leadership in this role. The visionary could also use this worksheet as a discussion tool.

Questions	*Notes*
What vision have you painted to inspire the partners and help them maintain focus on the goal?	
Has everyone bought into this vision? Is the original goal still valid? What are the possible areas of disagreement?	
Could the team measure and communicate progress better? How can you put the faces of those the project is trying to help in front of the partners?	

WORKSHEET FOR THE STRATEGIST: UPDATING THE STRATEGY

The strategist has the ability to see the big picture and the details simultaneously and to articulate the possible pathways to achieving the goal. The partner who assumes strategy leadership will need to monitor progress against that strategy/strategies constantly, to identify the need to follow the strategy more closely, or to change the strategy based on circumstances.

Major strategy/strategies	Progress toward strategy/ strategies	What needs to be changed?

DIAGNOSTIC WORKSHEET FOR THE TEAM BUILDER: DEVELOPING AN OPEN PARTNERSHIP CULTURE

The role of team builder involves helping the partners understand the various perspectives in the room and bridging those views in a way that aligns all partners behind the central goal. The person responsible for team building can use this worksheet to diagnose the culture of the partnership and develop ideas for gradually moving toward a more open culture, where members can problem-solve together (see Chapter 4).

Issue	How the issue applies to our partnership
Among our members, are there cultural differences across regions and countries?	
What are the cultural differences among the participating organizations (including governmental, nongovernmental, and private-sector organizations) and across such different sectors as health, education, finance, agriculture, and transportation?	
Which of these cultures characterizes each partner's organization: closed, synchronous, random, or open?	
What value does each culture represented provide to the team?	
What are the cultural differences among individuals, including values, style, knowledge, and self-interest?	
How can we move to a more open culture, in which participants work together to solve problems?	

WORKSHEET FOR THE TEAM BUILDER: MANAGING CONFLICT

In situations when two members of the group are in conflict, the team builder can use this tool to plan ways to manage the conflict. Methods may range from private discussions between the team builder and each individual to a three-way meeting facilitated by the team builder to coaching by an external consultant. This worksheet will help the team builder clarify the nature of the conflict and plan how to resolve it.

Steps	Questions	Conclusions
Diagnosis	Along the scale of assertiveness, where does each person lie?	
	Along the scale of cooperativeness, where does each person lie?	
Planning	What are the underlying concerns of each partner?	
	How can you convey the concerns of each partner to the other privately?	
	Is it likely the conflict can be lessened without a meeting of the two partners? If so, what steps can be taken?	
	If the conflict indicates a meeting is needed, what is the best way to bring the two partners together for a productive exchange?	
Facilitation (if needed)	What opening comments can you make to create a nonthreatening atmosphere and frame the importance of collaboration?	
	What will you ask each partner to convey to the other?	
	What specific request will you make to each partner for behavior in upcoming team meetings?	

WORKSHEET FOR THE ADVOCATE:
GETTING STAKEHOLDERS ON BOARD

Every partnership has a need for someone to play an advocacy role, a passion-ate spokesperson who can champion the cause externally and sway others to support the project's goal. In some cases advocacy is directed toward generating funds or services; in other cases the purpose is to bring NGOs and agencies on board. Regardless of the stakeholder group being targeted, a critical function of the advocate is to identify areas of mutual interests that form the basis for working together. The person who plays the advocate role can use this worksheet for planning stakeholder communication and interaction.

Stakeholder	Mission	Mutual interests	Opportunity to interact	Plan for action

WORKSHEET FOR THE POLITICAL INFLUENCER: GETTING OFFICIALS ON BOARD

Many partnerships have a need to influence government officials, whether the goal is funding, legislation, or behavioral change. Although the role is similar to the role of the advocate, the person who plays this role needs to have not only advocacy skills but also relationships among the targeted officials. The partner who takes responsibility for exerting political influence can use this worksheet to plan interactions between members of the partnership and government officials.

Targeted official	Opportunities for interacting	Partners to tap for interacting with officials

WORKSHEET FOR THE NETWORKER: LEVERAGING CONNECTIONS

The networker role calls for a leader who has already developed a large network of relationships across multiple sectors. This person is the one who can readily tap needed members for the partnership or open doors to talk with individuals who are key to carrying out the partnership's strategy. The networker can use this worksheet to plan ways to leverage both his or her connections and those of other partners.

Partner	Connections with potential influencers	Plans for interacting with influencers	Desired outcome

LEADERSHIP CHECKUP

This tool can serve as a discussion guide, to allow the partnership to reflect on how well the partners are filling leadership roles and what needs to be changed. All partners should participate in the discussion, not only the leaders.

	Poor	Good	Excellent
Sharing leadership			
How well are we filling gaps in leadership? Are all of the internal and external leadership functions being carried out?	❑	❑	❑
How well does the partnership's overall environment encourage people to voluntarily step up to leadership roles?	❑	❑	❑
How easily do people step down when their leadership role is no longer needed?	❑	❑	❑
How well are the leaders suppressing their egos and personal interests to work in the partnership's best interests?	❑	❑	❑
Convening			
How well are meetings planned?	❑	❑	❑
Is the facilitator able to create an open environment, in which all members participate?	❑	❑	❑
Is needed information being communicated before and after meetings?	❑	❑	❑
Are follow-up actions clarified at meetings and monitored afterward?	❑	❑	❑

	Poor	*Good*	*Excellent*
Communicating a vision			
Has one of the partners communicated a clear vision that other partners support?	❑	❑	❑
Do we have a clear goal and way(s) to measure progress against that vision?	❑	❑	❑
Shaping a strategy			
Is it clear how we will achieve the vision?	❑	❑	❑
Are changes needed in the strategy we have developed?	❑	❑	❑
Building a team			
Where are we along the spectrum of developing teamwork (recognition of differences, conflict, greater harmony, or accomplishment)?	❑	❑	❑
Are we becoming more cohesive?	❑	❑	❑
Advocating			
Do we have a partner with the ability to convey passion about our cause to external audiences or individuals?	❑	❑	❑
Is that partner actively serving as our spokesperson?	❑	❑	❑
Have we seen evidence that behaviors are changing as a result?	❑	❑	❑

	Poor	*Good*	*Excellent*
Achieving political influence			
Is one of our partners able to tap into the right government leaders at the right time?	❑	❑	❑
In what government area do we need to exert more influence?	❑	❑	❑
Networking			
Are we taking advantage of the full networking capabilities of our partner group?	❑	❑	❑
Do we have a plan for networking among key stakeholder groups?	❑	❑	❑

With the goal in sight and the imminent dissolution of the partnership just around the corner, several important exercises will enable a smooth transition and increase the likelihood of program sustainability once the partnership leaves it in the hands of local stakeholders.

THE LAST MILE: The Main Menu

Element	Tools
Adapting the approach to sustain momentum	Refocusing the approach to surveillance
	Involving local stakeholders
	Adapting and continuously improving the intervention strategy
Transferring control and giving credit	Transferring control checklist
	Worksheet for sharing credit
Capturing and communicating lessons learned	Partnership self-evaluation
	Identifying and communicating lessons learned
Dissolving the partnership	Discussion guide for partnership dissolution

REFOCUSING THE APPROACH TO SURVEILLANCE

In partnerships focused on intervention, a change in approach to surveillance is often needed in the Last Mile as the number of cases declines. While increasing capabilities to conduct surveillance earlier in a partnership typically lead to detection of a greater number of cases, the number of cases detected drops as a partnership nears its goal. At this point the partners must look harder for cases and use new tools to identify those cases and sort out the false positives they will encounter. With the smallpox eradication project, for example, the team shifted their surveillance strategy as the number of cases reported fell. They set up a reward system to encourage health workers to work harder to find cases. This worksheet may be helpful to partners in the Last Mile, as they consider whether changes are needed in their approach to surveillance.

Questions
_____

How do we need to change our methods of case finding, reporting, and analysis to keep up with the changes that have occurred?

What new tools and resources are needed?

What can we do to assure that surveillance continues even after active control measures have ended?

How can we draw the appropriate lessons from our experience?

INVOLVING LOCAL STAKEHOLDERS

Another way successful teams adapt to the needs of the Last Mile is to place greater emphasis on involving local stakeholders as the intervention spreads to additional communities. For example, it may be important to tie the partnership's program into the existing health system to ensure long-term sustainability and/or to rely on key local stakeholders to continue the program efforts after the partnership has left. To the extent that tasks change in the Last Mile (at a time when funding is running out), new partners and other resources from inside a country as well as outside may also be needed.

Questions

What new challenges do we face in completing our project?

Which local stakeholders could help us address those challenges?

How can we gain their support and commitment to reach the end goal of the partnership?

How can we tie our program into the other components of the health system, thereby strengthening the local health system?

ADAPTING AND CONTINUOUSLY IMPROVING INTERVENTION STRATEGY

Successful partnerships are continuously improving their strategy based on their experience to date. They are also alert to changes in the environment that may have strategic implications in the Last Mile. As more people receive treatment, for example, fewer cases appear in the population, and this change in the environment typically requires a change in strategy. The questions below may be helpful to teams in the Last Mile as they consider the need to adapt their strategy.

Questions

What lessons have we learned from our experience to date (and from the experience of others) that might help to improve our effort?

What new challenges are keeping us from accomplishing our goal?

How can we adapt our strategy to address those lessons and challenges?

What additional resources are required?

How will we measure our progress in the Last Mile?

TRANSFERRING CONTROL CHECKLIST

Successful partnerships must plan how they will transfer control of the project to regional and local leaders as soon as the team senses the Last Mile has begun. Given any changes in strategy that have been identified and additional stakeholders needed to support the changes, the team should clarify the roles that will have to be filled and who should fill them. The team must also find ways to gain their support, encourage ownership, identify constraints (financial, human resources, technological, and so on), and work with them to address the challenges ahead.

Role to be filled	Local stakeholder most appropriate for the role	Ways to encourage the stakeholder to take on responsibility

WORKSHEET FOR SHARING CREDIT

In an earlier part of the toolkit we provided a tool for sharing credit. This is particularly important as a project nears its end to ensure efforts will continue once the partnership is dissolved. It also creates support for future partnerships: by helping local stakeholders to celebrate the program's success locally, you increase the likelihood countries and communities will sustain the program and invest in future partnerships out of a sense of pride and ownership.

In addition, it is important for the partners to discuss what kind of recognition is needed by each of their organizations. Such recognition helps lay a foundation of trust and respect that encourages collaboration in future projects partners may have with each other. As several global health leaders have observed, "credit should be infinitely divisible." This worksheet can serve as a guide for partner discussion and a tool for planning.

Stakeholder/ partnering organization	Recognition needs	Opportunities for giving credit	Specific activities to give credit

1. *Stakeholder/partnering organization.* In this column partners should list the sponsoring organizations for the project and other key stakeholders.

2. *Recognition needs.* Each partner should speak candidly about how much and what kind of credit its organization will need to continue its support for the partnership. This could take the form of local media attention of success visible to a governing body. Partners should also discuss the needs of other stakeholders.

3. *Opportunities for giving credit.* This column can be used by the partners to identify outlets and opportunities to provide that credit.

4. *Specific activities to give credit.* Partners can brainstorm specific activities that will provide each partnering organization or other stakeholder with the appropriate form of credit. (More than one activity can apply to the same opportunity in the previous column.)

PARTNERSHIP SELF-EVALUATION

Before the dissolution of the partnership, it is important to evaluate how the partnership did in terms of reaching the goal and working as a team. This tool can serve as a guide for the discussion.

	Element	The degree to which the partnership succeeded	Major challenges	Lessons learned
First Mile checkup	Goal			
	Membership			
	Structure of partnership			
	Strategy of partnership			

	Element	The degree to which the partnership succeeded	Major challenges	Lessons learned
Management checkup	Research and planning			
	Launching, measuring, and communicating			
	Problem solving			
	Revising operating plan			
Leadership checkup	*Team leadership roles*			
	Convener			
	Visionary			
	Strategist			
	Team builder			
	External leadership roles			
	Advocate			
	Political influencer			
	Networker			

IDENTIFYING AND COMMUNICATING LESSONS LEARNED

Based on the results of the "Partnership Self-Evaluation," teams can use the tool below to identify and communicate lessons learned, both from successes and failures. It's particularly important to debrief failures so the team itself can learn from each mistake and can warn others before they make the same mistake. When debriefing failures, in particular, it is important to follow four steps:

1. Admit to making the mistake.
2. Learn from the mistake.
3. Warn others before they make the same mistake.
4. Get over the mistake and move on.

This worksheet provides a way to debrief projects and avoid future mistakes based on what did or did not work.

Aspect	Notes
Project to be debriefed	
Goals/objectives of project	
Team members and their roles	
Project time period	
Date and time of debriefing	

Aspect	Notes
What went well?	
What did not go well?	
Did we meet our goals? Why or why not?	
What did we learn from our successes?	
What did we learn from our failures?	
What would we do differently?	
What message would be valuable to spread to others so they could avoid our mistakes?	
What forum (for example, speech or workshop) or form of publication would be appropriate for communicating these lessons (Web or print)?	
Which partner(s) should be responsible for communicating these lessons?	

DISCUSSION GUIDE FOR PARTNERSHIP DISSOLUTION

When reaching the Last Mile, it is important for partners to think carefully about how to dissolve the partnership. Use the following questions to guide this conversation.

Questions

Has the partnership reached its goal?

What impact has the partnership had in the field of global health?

What, if any, value would be added if the partnership continued?

What loose ends (final communications, final credit giving, dissemination of lessons learned) need to be tied up?

What actions and what target date are appropriate to dissolve the partnership?

The Donor Toolkit

A pivotal force for ensuring that the lessons of collaboration are applied is the donor community—the global agencies, bilaterals, multilaterals, NGOs, foundations, and private-sector organizations that have made a commitment to global health. In every successful partnership we profiled, donors played a highly supportive role in providing strategic guidance, supporting local area infrastructure, and/or encouraging collaboration between members of a partnership. The following tools are examples of additional ways donors can support collaboration.

DONORS: THE MAIN MENU

Element	Tools
Leveraging grants to encourage collaboration	Statement of plans to incorporate collaborative practices
	Examples of impact measurement
	Developing a senior fellows program
Adapting policies to strengthen support for infrastructure	Recipient country feedback to donors
Supporting skill development in leadership and management	Supporting grantees with active learning
	Planning investment in a leadership center

Element	Tools
Sponsoring forums for leaders to reach consensus on priorities	Planning a priority forum on a specific disease or health threat
Modeling collaborative behaviors	Grantee feedback to donor

STATEMENT OF PLANS TO INCORPORATE COLLABORATIVE PRACTICES

The heart of close collaboration is the partner group itself—the individuals who arrive with different perspectives to try to reach a single goal. Whether they will become a team that can share ideas openly and solve problems together hangs in the balance when they meet for the first time. Donors can help disseminate the lessons for making that happen by adopting grant policies that hold recipients accountable for effective collaboration practices. For example, donors can require an explicit statement from partnerships about how collaboration will occur over the course of the project. This worksheet will help them develop this statement.

Questions

How will the partners work with each other?

How will the partnership provide for feedback from individual partners?

How will resources be used to support meetings and other means of communication between partners?

(as applicable) How will the partners work with the ministries of health and finance in countries being served? How will the partners identify other relevant ministries and stakeholders and work with them? How will the partners encourage the relevant stakeholders to work together?

WORKSHEET: EXAMPLES OF IMPACT MEASUREMENT

As we described in Chapter 7, global health leaders are only beginning to learn how to measure their progress in terms of impact rather than process. Our advisory group suggested that donors work closely with potential grant recipients to help them design an effective way to evaluate their efforts—for example, providing potential partnerships with examples of how teams have measured progress in similar efforts (drawing from outside as well as inside global health). Donors can use this worksheet to develop a list of examples that illustrate good practices they would like to see applied.

Type of partnership	Name of partnership	Goal	Impact measurement
Advocacy			
Research			
Intervention			
Technology exchange			
Policy development			
Other			

WORKSHEET: DEVELOPING A SENIOR FELLOWS PROGRAM

Leaders in global health suggested that donors develop a cadre of senior fellows from all sectors who are experienced in global health and willing to work on-site with partnerships at critical stages in a project. These questions are designed to guide a discussion among the donor's senior team, to determine how a fellows program might be developed. The questions can be distributed in advance and summarized before the meeting to spark discussion.

How can we identify potential fellows? What sectors should we include? Which of our previous grantees have been particularly successful in building collaborative partnerships?

What will we ask them to do?

How will we communicate the availability of fellows to partnerships in each sector?

What administrative support will we provide? Will we cover expenses of fellows, or will that be expensed to the partnerships?

How will we assess the impact of the fellows program?

RECIPIENT COUNTRY FEEDBACK TO DONOR

In our research we heard repeatedly that the "voice of the South" should be heard to a greater extent. We also heard that to get truly constructive feedback, donors need to work hard to overcome the grantees' fear that criticizing donors will cause the donors to withdraw their support. One means of hearing this voice and encouraging honesty is to develop a method of gathering feedback from program recipients. The following is a list of questions that might be used to gather such feedback.

Which of the following characteristics are most important for donors (please check)?

☐ Understanding local culture

☐ Communicating effectively with political leaders and communities

☐ Providing training for health workers and volunteers

☐ Investing in health systems

☐ Providing substantial resources

☐ Demonstrating ongoing interest in the country

☐ Other _____

Of the donors who have sponsored efforts in your country, which five come closest to having these characteristics?

1. _____
2. _____
3. _____
4. _____
5. _____

Which are the top three diseases/threats in your country, in order of importance?

1. _____
2. _____
3. _____

Of these, which diseases/threats are not being addressed adequately?

1. _____
2. _____
3. _____

Do you have the capacity within your infrastructure to integrate the goals and coordinate the programs of different donors? How could donors help strengthen this capacity?

Which of these infrastructure capabilities are most needed in your country (circle needs)? How could donors address each of them (fill in response)? Financial skills:

Management skills:

Monitoring systems:

Laboratories:

Public health workers:

WORKSHEET: PROVIDING ACTIVE LEARNING TO GRANTEES

Effective collaboration can be taught, but it requires active learning and ongoing coaching. Donors are in an excellent position to connect their grantees with the individuals and organizations that can provide skill building in collaboration that goes beyond simply understanding a particular set of principles or guidelines, to active learning—providing instruction and guidance as the grantees actually struggle in real time with building, strengthening, and maintaining their partnership. The questions below are designed to guide a discussion among the donor's senior team members about how they might develop such an effort.

Questions

How can we identify those grant programs that would benefit from active learning? What are the criteria we will use to select the grantees for whom this is appropriate?

How can we identify partnerships that would benefit from being grouped together and sharing their experience in a common active learning "collaborative?"

Who are the individuals and institutions that could provide this active learning? What process or mechanism do we use to ensure it takes place?

How can we measure the value added by active learning?

Should we structure this into grants?

WORKSHEET: PLANNING INVESTMENT IN A LEADERSHIP CENTER

Donors can encourage the development of leadership and management skills by providing support for NGOs and institutions that express an interest in the area. For example, donors might endow chairs at universities, fund fellowships at NGOs or successful partnerships, invest in centers of leadership, or fund the development of case materials for leadership and management, based on successful collaborations. These questions are designed to guide a discussion among the donor's senior team, to determine how a leadership center might be developed. The questions can be distributed in advance and summarized before the meeting to spark discussion.

How could a leadership center help us achieve our mission?

What institutions are now providing leadership training that is appropriate for or could be adapted to global health?

Which individuals and institutions could provide the best leadership and environment for the center?

What steps should we take to explore the possibility of starting a center?

WORKSHEET: PLANNING A PRIORITY FORUM ON A SPECIFIC DISEASE/THREAT

Leaders in global health have suggested that donors bring together those leaders who are working on a particular disease/threat, so they can reach consensus about the best ways to coordinate efforts. For example, a donor or donors might sponsor a retreat, let people present where we are and lessons learned, and analyze what is needed and the best way to get there (including the goal of each priority and potential partnerships that could be formed). For such discussions, it's very important to have a mixture of people— Americans and non-Americans, developing country leaders and developed country leaders. If the forum is sponsored by a single donor, that donor can then use the results of the forum to shape its own grant-making agenda.

These questions below are designed to guide a discussion among a donor's senior team, to determine how a priority forum might be developed. The questions can be distributed in advance and summarized before the meeting to spark discussion.

What are the problem areas for which this sort of forum would be useful?

What sectors should we include? Who are the key players currently in this field, including donors, multinational organizations, NGOs, the private sector, and national governments? Who are the other stakeholders that should be invited?

What are the lessons we can learn from what has been done to date?

Do we want to solicit input widely by e-mail or phone calls before the forum assembles? How can the agenda be structured to emphasize discussions rather than presentations? Who should facilitate the forum?

How will we assess the impact of the forum in terms of improving collaborative outcomes?

GRANTEE FEEDBACK TO DONOR

Many of those we interviewed suggested that donors serve as models for collaborative behavior, strengthening their capacity to work with their own organizational units and with external partners. For example, donors can use a tool such as the following to determine how well they encourage collaboration among partners who have received a grant.

Questions

Which of the following collaborative practices does our donor organization follow with other donors (please check)?
- ☐ Takes only joint credit when funding joint projects with other donors
- ☐ Works in tandem with other donors within a country
- ☐ Sponsors training in collaboration, in conjunction with other donor organizations
- ☐ Listens closely to what is said
- ☐ Provides for long-term sustainability of the project

Which of the following collaborative practices did our donor organization follow with your partnership? (please check)
- ☐ Provided a workshop to train partners in collaborative practices as the project began
- ☐ Required feedback by individual partners about how well the partners were collaborating
- ☐ Included resources dedicated to communication between partners, including meetings, phone conferences, and other means of communication
- ☐ Initiated discussion with leaders of your partnership about how to make the program sustainable

What suggestions do you have for improvement? Are there ways that the administrative and procedural requirements of the donor could be changed to facilitate collaboration?

Appendix I. *Coalitions and Collaboration in Global Health:*
A Dialogue Hosted by the Task Force for Global Health
(formerly the Task Force for Child Survival and Development)

LIST OF PARTICIPANTS

This dialogue among global health leaders took place on November 10–11, 2005, in Atlanta, Georgia.

Seth Berkley, MD, president and CEO, International AIDS Vaccine Initative

Stephen Blount, MD, director, Coordinating Office of Global Health, Centers for Disease Control and Prevention (CDC)

George F. Brown, MD, MPH, director, Health Equity, Rockefeller Foundation

Kathy Cahill, MPH, senior program officer, Bill & Melinda Gates Foundation

Lincoln Chen, MD, MPH, director, Global Equity Initative

Ernest Darkoh, MD, MPH, MBA, chair, BroadReach Healthcare, LLC

Louis de Merode, MS, MA, principal, Silver Creek Associates

Walter R. Dowdle, PhD, senior consultant to WHO, Polio Eradication Program, The Task Force for Child Survival and Development

Michael Eriksen, ScD, professor and director, Institute of Public Health, Georgia State University

Bill Foege, MD, MPH, senior adviser, Bill & Melinda Gates Foundation

John Hardman, MD, executive director, The Carter Center

Farnoosh Hashemian, MPH, research associate, Department of Global Health, School of Public Health, Yale University

Elisabeth Hayes, MBA, senior program associate, The Task Force for Child Survival and Development

Jacob Kumaresan, MD, PhD, MPH, president, International Trachoma Initiative

Margaret McIntyre, MBA, senior associate director, Global Road Safety Forum, The Task Force for Child Survival and Development

Michael Merson, MD, Anna M. R. Lauder Professor of Public Health, School of Public Health, Yale University

Nancy Neill, MA, founder, Atlanta Communications Group, LLC

Eric Ottesen, MD, director, Lymphatic Filariasis Support Center, The Task Force for Child Survival and Development

Mark Rosenberg, MD, MPP, executive director, The Task Force for Child Survival and Development

Dave Ross, ScD, director, Public Health Informatics Institute, The Task Force for Child Survival and Development

Ian Smith, MD, adviser to the director-general, World Health Organization

Anil Soni, director, Pharmaceutical Services, Clinton Foundation HIV/AIDS Initiative

Michael St. Louis, MD, chief science officer, Coordinating Office for Global Health, CDC

Nana Twum-Danso, MD, MPH, associate director, Mectizan Donation Program, The Task Force for Child Survival and Development

Pascal Villeneuve, MD, chief, Health Section, Programme Division, UNICEF

Appendix 2. *Coalitions and Collaboration in Global Health: A Symposium for Global Health Leaders*

LIST OF PARTICIPANTS

The symposium took place on October 19–20, 2006, at the Carter Center in Atlanta, Georgia.

Samira Asma, DDS, MPH, associate director, Global Tobacco Control, Office of Smoking and Health, National Center for Chronic Disease Prevention and Health Promotion, Centers for Disease Control and Prevention (CDC)

Ramadan Assi, Presidential Scholar (AED), Rollins School of Public Health

Mir Omar Atefi, MD, Humphrey Fellow, Rollins School of Public Health

James Austin, DBA, MBA, professor, general management, Harvard Business School

Anna Awimbo, research director, Microcredit Summit Campaign

Edward L. Baker Jr., MD, MPH, MSc, director, North Carolina Institute for Public Health

Victor Barnes, PhD, MA, director, HIV/AIDS Programs, Corporate Council for Africa

Seth Berkley, MD, president and CEO, International AIDS Vaccine Initative

Donald Berwick, MD, MPP, president and CEO, Institute for Healthcare Improvement

Martha Bidez, PhD, president and CEO, Bidez & Associates

Barry Bloom, PhD, ScD, AM, dean of the faculty of public health, Harvard University School of Public Health

Stephen Blount, MD, director, Coordinating Office of Global Health, CDC

Thomas H. Bornemann, EdD, director, Mental Health Programs, Carter Center

Senkham Boutdara, MD, Humphrey Fellow, Rollins School of Public Health

George F. Brown, MD, MPH, consultant, Hewlett Foundation

Peter Brown, PhD, MA, professor, director, Global Water Initiative, Emory University

Ghada Bsiki, MD, Humphrey Fellow, Rollins School of Public Health

Scott Burris, JD, professor, Temple University Beasley School of Law

President Jimmy Carter, founder, The Carter Center

Michael Conway, JD, partner, Global Public Health Practice, McKinsey & Company

Alan Court, director, Programme Division, UNICEF

James W. Curran, MD, MPH, dean, Rollins School of Public Health, Emory University

Nils Daulaire, MD, MPH, president and CEO, Global Health Council

Walter R. Dowdle, PhD, senior consultant to WHO, Polio Eradication Program

Michael Eriksen, ScD, professor and director, Institute of Public Health

John Evans, MD, chair, MaRS Discovery District

Henry Falk, MD, MPH, director, Coordinating Center for Environmental Health and Injury Prevention, CDC

Armin Fidler, MD, MPH, MSc, health sector manager, Europe and Central Asia Region, World Bank

Bill Foege, MD, MPH, senior adviser, Bill & Melinda Gates Foundation

Daniel M. Fox, PhD, president, Milbank Memorial Fund

Justine Frain, PhD, vice president, Global Community Partnerships, Glaxo Smith Kline

Helene Gayle, MD, MPH, president and CEO, CARE

William H. Gimson III, MBA, chief operating officer, CDC

Roger I. Glass, MD, PhD, associate director, International Programs, National Institutes of Health

Howard Goldberg, PhD, associate director, Global Health, Division of Reproductive Health

David Green, founder and executive director, Project Impact, Inc.

Thandeka Gugu Gcaba, Humphrey Fellow, Rollins School of Public Health

Anu Gupta, corporate contributions, Johnson & Johnson

Rajesh Gupta, MD/MS candidate, Stanford University

Andy Haines, MBBS, MD, FRCGP, FFPHM, FRCP, FMedSci, director, London School of Hygiene and Tropical Medicine

Elisabeth Hayes, MBA, assistant program director, The Task Force for Child Survival and Development

Rafe Henderson, MD, MPH, MPP, former assistant director-general, World Health Organization

David Heymann, MD, DTM&H, representative of the director-general, Polio Eradication, assistant director-general, Communicable Diseases, World Health Organization

Howard Hiatt, MD, professor of medicine, Harvard Medical School and senior physician

Alan Hinman, MD, MPH, senior public health scientist, Public Health Informatics Institute, The Task Force for Child Survival and Development

Karen Hofman, MD, director, Division of Advanced Studies and Policy Analysis, National Institutes of Health

Susan E. Holck, MD, general management, World Health Organization

Donald Hopkins, MD, MPH, associate executive director, Carter Center

Richard Keenlyside, associate director for science, Global AIDS Program, National Center for HIV/AIDS, Viral Hepatitis, STD, and TB Prevention

Alison Kelly, strategy and innovation officer, Coordinating Office for Global Health (COGH), CDC

Ali S. Khan, MD, MPH, acting deputy director, National Center for Zoonotic, Vector Borne, and Enteric Diseases, CDC

Jim Kim, MD, PhD, director, HIV/AIDS, World Health Organization

Irene Koek, MA, division chief, Infectious Diseases, Bureau for Global Health, USAID

Sudha Rani Kotha, JD, MPH, deputy director, Global Health Programs, University of Michigan School of Public Health

Stephen Lewis, special envoy, HIV/AIDS in Africa, United Nations

Adetokunbo Lucas, MD, professor of international health, Harvard University

Vincent Maku, MS, Humphrey Fellow, Rollins School of Public Health

Chad Martin, MPH, deputy strategy and innovation officer, COGH, CDC

Boiketho Matshalaga, Foege Fellow, Rollins School of Public Health

Joe McCannon, vice president, Institute for Healthcare Improvement

Deborah McFarland, PhD, MSc, MPH, professor, Global Health, Rollins School of Public Health

Sarah McKune, MPH, consultant

Michael Merson, MD, Anna M. R. Lauder Professor of Public Health, Yale University, School of Public Health

Stephen Morrison, PhD, executive director, HIV/AIDS Task Force; director, Africa Program, Center for Strategic and International Studies

Deborah E. Myers, MA, director, External and Government Affairs and Public Partnerships, GlaxoSmithKline Biologicals

Nancy Neill, MA, consultant, Atlanta Communications Group

Eric Ottesen, MD, director, Lymphatic Filariasis Support Center, The Task Force for Child Survival and Development

Ariel Pablos Mendez, MD, MPH, director, Knowledge Management and Sharing, World Health Organization

David Ray, MA, director, Constituency Building, CARE USA

Mark L. Rosenberg, MD, executive director, The Task Force for Child Survival and Development

David Ross, ScD, director, Public Health Informatics Institute, The Task Force for Child Survival and Development

Louis Rowitz, PhD, professor, Community Health Sciences, School of Public Health, University of Illinois at Chicago

Kristin Saarlas, MPH, deputy director, Public Health Informatics Institute

Dieudonne Sankara, MD, Foege Fellow, Rollins School of Public Health

David J. Sencer, MD, MPH, former director, CDC

Michel Sidibé, director, Country and Regional Support, UNAIDS

Patricia Simone, MD, director, Division of Epidemiology and Surveillance Capacity Development, Coordinating Office for Global Health

Sanjay Sinho, MD, MA, health unit director, CARE

Ian M. Smith, MD, advisor to the director-general, World Health Organization

Anil Soni, director, Pharmaceutical Services, Clinton Foundation HIV/AIDS Initiative

Katerina Spasovska, MD, MS, Humphrey Fellow, Rollins School of Public Health

Michael St. Louis, MD, science officer, COGH, CDC

Richard Stanley, director, Richard Stanley Productions

Kari Stoever, RN, senior program manager, Albert B. Sabin Vaccine Institute

Jeffrey L. Sturchio, MD, vice president, External Affairs, Human Health-Europe, Middle East, Africa, and Canada, Merck and Co., Inc.

Bjorn Thylefors, MD, director, Mectizan Donation Program

Landry Tsague, MD, Foege Fellow, Rollins School of Public Health

Nana Twum-Danso, MD, MPH, director, Mebendazole Donation Initiative

Pascal Villeneuve, MD, chief, Health Section, Programme Division, UNICEF

Bill Watson, former deputy director, COC, and co-founder, The Task Force for Child Survival and Development

Ellen Wild, MPH, director of programs, Public Health Informatics Institute

Paul Zeitz, DO, MPH, executive director, Global AIDS Alliance

Paul Zintl, MD, chief operating officer, Partners in Health

WORKS CITED

Acharya, Tara, Charles A. Gardner, and Derek Yach. *Technological Innovation, Social Innovation, and the Role of Developing Countries in Global Health.* Health affairs (Project Hope), 2007; 26(4): 1052–61.

Amazigo, Uche. "Twenty Years of Mectizan Mass Treatment." Mectizan Donation Program, Decatur, Ga., 2007.

Austin, James E., Ezequiel Reficco, and Gabriel Berger. *Social Partnering in Latin America: Lessons Drawn from Collaborations of Businesses and Civil Society Organizations.* David Rockefeller Center Series on Latin American Studies. Cambridge: Harvard University Press, 2004.

Benton, B., J. Bump, A. Sékétéli, and B. Liese. "Partnership and Promise: Evolution of the African River Blindness Campaigns." *Annals of Tropical Medicine and Parasitology* 96, supplement 1 (March 2002): 5–14 (10).

Bill & Melinda Gates Foundation. *Developing Successful Global Health Alliances.* April 2002. Available online at http://www.gatesfoundation.org/nr/downloads/globalhealth/GlobalHealthAlliances.pdf.

Bowles, Newton. *The Task Force for Child Survival and Development: Hope as Energy: An Experiment, 1984–1998.* New York: UNICEF, 1998.

Caines, Karen. *Assessing the Impact of Global Health Partnerships.* London: Department for International Development (DFID) Health Resource Center, 2004.

Collins, James C. *Good to Great and the Social Sectors: Why Business Thinking Is Not the Answer.* New York: HarperCollins, 2005.

Curran, Jim. *K2: Triumph and Tragedy.* Boston: Houghton Mifflin, 1989.

De Quadros, Ciro. "On toward Victory." In *Polio.* Edited by Thomas M. Daniel and Frederick C. Robinson, 182–98. New York: University of Rochester Press, 1997.

Etheridge, Elizabeth W. *Sentinel for Health: A History of the Centers for Disease Control.* Berkeley: University of California Press, 1992.

Filerman, Gary L., and Clarence E. Pearson. "The Mandate: Transformational Leadership." In *Critical Issues in Global Health.* Edited by E. Jossey, E. Koop, C. E. Pearson, and M. R. Schwarz, 446–54. San Francisco: Jossey-Bass, 2002.

Foege, William F. "Health Ministers as Good Ancestors?" Address delivered at the Fifty-third World Health Assembly. May 16, 2000. Available online at http://ftp.who.int/gb/archive/pdf_files/WHA53/ead6.pdf.

——— et al., eds. *Global Health Leadership and Management.* San Francisco: Jossey-Bass, 2005.

———, Nils Daulaire, Robert E. Black, and Clarence E. Pearson. "A New Role for Corporate America." In *Global Health Leadership and Management.* Edited by William F. Foege et al., 9–24. San Francisco: Jossey-Bass, 2005.

Frost, Laura, Michael R. Reich, and Tomoko Fujisaki. "A Partnership for Ivermectin: Social Worlds and Boundary Objects." In *Public-Private Partnerships for Public Health.* Edited by Michael R. Reich. Cambridge: Harvard Center for Population and Development Studies, distributed by Harvard University Press, 2002.

Fujimura, Sara Francis. "The Man Who Made Polio History." *Perspectives in Health* 10, no. 2 (2005): 10–14. Available online at http://www.paho.org/English/dd/pin/perspectives22.pdf.

Gerberding, Julie. "The Main Way to Stop AIDS—Strategies That Put Prevention First Will Ease Disease's Toll." *Atlanta Journal Constitution,* June 12, 2006, A15.

Greenleaf, Robert K. *The Servant as Leader.* Indianapolis, Ind.: Robert K. Greenleaf Center, 1970.

Gupta, Rajat K., and Lynn Taliento. "How Businesses Can Combat Global Disease." *McKinsey Quarterly* (December 2003): 100–3.

Hofstede, Gert, and Gert Jan Hofstede. *Cultures and Organizations: Software of the Mind.* Maidenhead, United Kingdom: McGraw Hill, 2005.

International Federation of Red Cross (IFRC) and Red Crescent Societies. *World Disasters Report 2005: Focus on Information in Disasters.* Geneva: IFRC, 2005.

Kagan, Sharon. *United We Stand.* New York: Teachers College Press, 1991.

Kantor, David, and William Lehr. *Inside the Family.* San Francisco: Jossey-Bass, 1975.

Kaplan, Robert S., and David P. Norton. "The Balanced Scorecard—Measures

That Drive Performance." *Harvard Business Review* (January–February 1992): 71–79.

Katzenbach, Jon R., and Douglas K. Smith. *The Wisdom of Teams.* Cambridge: Harvard Business School Press, 1993.

Keirsey, David, and Bates, Marilyn. *Please Understand Me: Character and Temperament Types.* Del Mar, Calif.: Prometheus Nemesis Books, 1984.

Levine, Ruth. *Millions Saved: Proven Successes in Global Health.* Washington, D.C.: Center for Global Development, 2004.

Linden, Russell M. *Working across Boundaries: Making Collaboration Work in Government and Nonprofit Organizations.* San Francisco: Jossey-Bass, 2002.

———. "How Businesses Can Combat Global Disease." Special Edition: Global Directions. *McKinsey Quarterly* (December 2003): 102.

Merson, Michael. "The HIV-AIDS Pandemic at Year Twenty-five—The Global Response," *New England Journal of Medicine* 354, no. 23 (June 2006): 2414–17.

Merson, Michael H., Robert E. Black, and Anne J. Mills. "Global Cooperation in International Public Health." In *International Public Health: Diseases, Programs, Systems, and Policies.* Edited by Michael H. Merson, Robert E. Black, and Anne J. Mills, 640–56. Gaithersburg, Md.: Aspen Publishers, 2001.

———. "Global Influence and Global Responses: International Health at the Turn of the Twenty-first Century." In *International Public Health: Diseases, Programs, Systems, and Policies.* Edited by Michael H. Merson, Robert E. Black, and Anne J. Mills. Gaithersburg, Md.: Aspen Publishers, 2001.

———, eds. *International Public Health: Diseases, Programs, Systems, and Policies.* Gaithersburg, Md.: Aspen Publishers, 2001.

Nankin, Jesse. "Prevention: It Just Makes Cents." *Harvard Public Health Review* (Spring–Summer 2007): 1–2.

Olson, Kate, and T. George Harris. "Defining Common Work: A Conversation with Rob Lehman." *Our Common Work* (Summer 2007).

Pigman, Herbert A. *Conquering Polio.* Evanston, Ill.: Rotary International, 2005.

Sauffman, Stuart A. *The Competitiveness of Nations in a Global Knowledge-based Economy.* Oxford: Oxford University Press, 2000.

"Smallpox Eradication: Memories and Milestones," *CDC Connects*, October 26, 2007, 5.

Smith, Raymond A., ed. *Encyclopedia of AIDS: A Social, Political, Cultural, and Scientific Record of the HIV Epidemic.* Chicago: Fitzroy Dearborn Pub-

lishers, 1998. Available online at http://www.thebody.com/content/
art14017.html.

UNAIDS. *2004 Report on the Global AIDS Epidemic: Fourth Global Report.*
Geneva: Joint United Nations Program on HIV/AIDS, 2004. Available
online at http://www.unaids.org/bangkok2004/report.html.

United Nations Development Program (UNDP). *Human Development Report
2007–2008.* New York: UNDP, 2008.

UN Africa Recovery from UNAIDS. World Bank data.

World Bank. *Addressing the Challenges of Globalization: An Independent Evaluation of the World Bank's Approach to Global Programs.* Washington, D.C.:
World Bank, 2004.

———. *Healthy Development: The World Bank Strategy for Health, Nutrition,
and Population Results.* Washington, D.C.: World Bank, 2007. Available
online at http://www.loc.gov/catdir/toc/ecip0719/2007022159.html.

———. *Synopsis of World Development Reports (1995–2005).* Washington, D.C.:
World Bank, 2006.

———. *World Development Indicators 1997.* Washington, D.C.: World Bank,
1997.

———. *World Development Indicators 2002.* Washington, D.C.: World Bank,
2002.

World Health Organization and World Bank. *World Report on Road Traffic
Injury Prevention.* Geneva: World Health Organization, 2004.

Accelerated Development and Intro-
    duction Plans (ADIPS), 47
accountability, lack of, 55–56
Acharya, Tara, 166
active learning, 169
adjacent possible, 63
advocacy partnerships, general, 88–89
advocate (external leadership role),
    137–38, 217
Africa, 113. *See also specific topics*
African Program for Onchocerciasis
    Control (APOC), 2, 58, 113, 114,
    122–25; approach to delivering
    Mectizan, 115–16
AIDS. *See* HIV/AIDS
Al-Hinai, Fuad Mubarak, 135–36,
    138–40
Al-Kharusi, Wahid, 130, 138, 141
anthrax scares, 120
Austin, James E., 64, 122, 146, 150,
    151, 154, 168
authority, 91

Baker, Ed, 142
Berkley, Seth, 27–28, 91, 92, 112, 135,
    163, 165
Berwick, Don, 89, 119, 121–22, 152

bilaterals, 28
Bill & Melinda Gates Foundation
    (Gates Foundation), 3–4, 28, 71, 75;
    report encouraging disciplined
    management, 108–9
Bliss, Tony, 133, 139, 140
Bone and Joint Decade (BJD), 130
Botswana, 45, 47
Bowles, Newton, 48, 86, 93, 94, 97–
    98, 100, 104
Browner, Bruce, 130
Buffet, Warren, 28
Burris, Scott, 171
Buse, Kent, 24
business, bias against, 55

Cahill, Kathy, 128, 136
Caines, Karen, 134
Carter, Jimmy, 12, 119, 170
Carter Center, 119
Center for Global Health Collabora-
    tion, 169
Centers for Disease Control (CDC),
    76t
Central Africa, 113
charter, topics to include in, 194–95

citizens, local: increased participation of, 22–23

Clinton Foundation, 7

close collaboration, 5f, 6t, 9; governance models relevant to, 95, 96t, 97–98; between individuals, 5f; research on, 9–12; success and, 4–9

closed (organizational) culture, 59, 60, 61t

collaboration: definitions, 9; increased importance and difficulty of, 29–30; laying foundations for, 12–13; Rob Lehman on, 7; statements about how it will occur over course of project, 161; ways donors can encourage, 13, 157–74, 160f; why it is top-of-mind for leaders in the field, 19–30. See also real collaboration, 9. See also close collaboration; specific topics

collaborative behaviors, modeling, 172–74

collaborative practices, statement of plans to incorporate, 234, 234t

collaborative team development, phases of, 134, 135f

Collins, Jim, 131

Coll-Seck, Awa Marie, 89–90, 102, 103, 137

communicating lessons learned, 152–54, 230–31t

communicating progress, 118–19

communication: among partners, 78–79, 122–23. See also under road-traffic injuries

Communications Plan Template, 203, 204t, 205

community-based programs, 115

community-directed treatment, 116

convener (team leadership role), 131–32, 212

Conway, Gordon, 173

Conway, Michael, 27, 154, 171

cooperation, 5f, 6t, 7

coordination, 5f, 6t

credit: giving, 151–52; sharing, 118, 205–6, 227–28

cultural differences: across countries and regions, 54–57; between partners, 52–54

culture: of global health, "mitigated," 102. See also organizational cultures

Curran, Jim, 42, 69, 77, 83n1, 85, 108, 127, 143

data collection, standardizing, 166–67

Daulaire, Nils, 111, 124, 141, 171

Davidson, Lucy, 94, 153–54

de Merode, Louis, 79

de Quadros, Ciro, 147–48

decision-making protocol, worksheet for, 186–87

Department for International Development (DFID), 3–4

developing countries: greater attention to global health, 20–21, 23t; minimizing reporting burden on, 164

development assistance for health, 20, 21f

disease/threat: challenges in dealing with, 41–45, 43t, 46t, 47–50; nature of, and response, 46t; stages of evolution of efforts to deal with, 34–50, 35f. See also specific topics

donor coordination conferences, 170–71

donor reports, key, 3–4

Donor Toolkit, 233–34t; statement of plans to incorporate collaborative practices, 234, 234t

donor watch, creating a, 172–73

donors: feedback to, 236, 237–38t, 241–42t; roles outside the funding arena, 159–60; ways to encourage collaboration, 13, 157–74, 160f

emotional intelligence (EQ), 91
Etheridge, Elizabeth, 149–50

Farmer, Paul, 71, 80
Fidler, Armin, 173
Filerman, Gary L., 139
First Mile, 85–87, 87f, 161–62; choosing the right membership, 73, 88–93; clarifying organizational roles, 75–76, 102–5; developing a shared goal, 73–74, 93–95; donors and, 13; elements that contribute to success, 72–76, 72f; laying foundations for collaboration in, 12–13; overall governance models, 95, 96t, 97–98; selecting an appropriate structure, 74–75, 95–98; shaping a big-picture strategy, 75, 98–102; tasks to focus on in, 13
First Mile Toolkit, 179–95
Foege, William H., 10; AIDS and, 33; Alan Hinman on, 131; on changing strategy, 151; on commitment to real collaboration, 12; on communicating success to stakeholders, 118; convener role and, 131; D. A. Henderson and, 155; on discipline in research and planning, 111; on donors encouraging collaboration, 163; on evaluation standards for grantees, 161; as executive director of Task Force, 87, 97; Gates Foundation and, 20, 22, 71; and Genesis of Task Force, 86; giving credit to in-country partners, 152; *Global Health Leadership and Management*, 20; on impact of Task Force's

strategy, 101; on infrastructure, 165; on management skills, 109; on onchocerciasis, 52; on optimism *vs.* cynicism, 91; PARTNERS and, 71; on partnerships defining goals, 73–74; personality, 131; polio program and, 147; positions held, 10, 20, 87, 97; Rafe Henderson on, 131; on size of partnership, 92–93; smallpox eradication program and, 143–46, 150, 152, 154

Gardner, Charles A., 166
Gates Foundation. *See* Bill & Melinda Gates Foundation
Gautam, Kul, 130
Gayle, Helene, 62
Gerberding, Julie, 33
Gilmartin, Raymond V., 22, 113–15, 163
GlaxoSmithKline (GSK), 58
Global Alliance for Vaccines and Immunization (GAVI), 2, 47
Global Alliance to Eliminate Lymphatic Filariasis, 59
Global Fund to Fight AIDS, Tuberculosis, and Malaria (Global Fund), 23, 83
global health: new expectations in, 19–23; traditional culture of, 54–56; what we have *vs.* what we need in, 29t, 30. *See also specific topics*
global health efforts, complex forces at play in, 13
Global Health Leadership and Management (Foege et al.), 20
global health partnerships (GHPs), 3–4; circumstances faced by, 34; conducting interventions, 89–90; degree of partnership integration, 5, 5f; effectiveness, 3–4; Genesis of, 70–72; options for missions of,

global health partnerships (continued)
37–41; purpose, 73 (see also goals);
structural models common to, 95,
96t, 97–98; supporting structures,
98. See also specific topics
global health sector, fundamental
shifts in architecture of, 23–24, 25f,
26–29
Global Polio Eradication Initiative
(GPEI), 123, 158, 159; organizational
roles in, 103, 103t
Global Road Safety Crisis: We Should
Do Much More, The, 141
Global Road Safety Forum, 141
Global Road Safety Steering Committee (GRS SC): advocacy task,
137; critical team leadership roles
and, 129–34, 136, 136t; policymaking and, 48–49; UN General
Assembly and, 41, 44, 137–39
globalization, 24
goal statements, worksheet for developing, 183–85
goals (of partnerships): activities that
can help partners develop, 94;
alignment of personal agendas
with, 90–91; measuring progress
toward, 116–18, 117f, 161. See also
shared goal
governance models, 95, 96t, 97–98
government agencies, sense of turf
among, 55
Grant, James, 2, 86, 95, 98
grant requirements, standardizing, 164
grantees: feedback to donor, 241–42t;
providing active learning to,
238–39t
grants: flexibility within, 162; leveraging to encourage collaboration,
160–63
Green Light Committee (GLC), 75,
82, 83

Guinea Worm Eradication Program
(GWEP), 117–19, 149
Gupta, Anu, 172
Gupta, Rajat K., 47

Hardman, John, 88–89
health, global. See global health
health equity, 22
"health for all" approach, 22
health monitoring and evaluation
systems: incorporating into projects, 165–66
health sector reform, 21–22
health spending increases in developing countries, 20–21, 23t
Henderson, D. A., 155
Henderson, Ralph ("Rafe"), 86, 116, 131
Heymann, David, 103
Hiatt, Howard, 71
highly active antiretroviral therapy
(HAART), 38
Hinman, Alan: on building political
will, 36; on collaboration, 87, 97;
on communication among partners, 78–79; on Foege, 131; on
infrastructure, 166; on Jim Grant,
98; on need for a visionary, 132; on
PARTNERS, 77; on productive
meetings, 122; Task Force and, 87;
on team members working together, 141
HIV/AIDS, 164, 170; Clinton Foundation and, 7; drug companies and,
7; drugs for, 32, 33, 38; evolution of
global health efforts to address,
37–39, 39f, 41–48, 42t; global
experience with, following technological advances, 32–34; policymaking efforts and, 49; prevention,
33–34; in Tanzania, 26f; threshold
in treatment, 38–39; vaccine for,
31–33, 112

HIV/AIDS patients in Lesotho, treatment of, 82

Hofstede, Geert, 56

Holck, Susan, 49, 134, 165

Hopkins, Don, 38, 117, 118, 149, 150–51

hub and spoke with secretariat (governance model), 96t

immunization. *See* vaccinations

individuals, differences in, 61–64

influence, 91. *See also* political influencer

informal organization (governance model), 96t

infrastructure, adapting policies to strengthen support for, 164–67

integrated team. *See* close collaboration

interactions, ground rules for, 192–93

Inter-Agency Coordinating Committee (ICC), 147, 148

International AIDS Vaccine Initiative (IAVI), 111, 165

International Development, Department for. *See* Department for International Development

International Public Health (Merson et al.), 24

Internet, 24

Journey, 13, 76–80, 79f; applying discipline in research and planning, 111–14; communicating progress, 118–19; complementary leadership roles, 127–42, 128f; discipline and flexibility in management, 78–79, 108–25, 110f; engaging partners in problem solving, 119–23; launching (the program), 114–16, 115t; measuring progress, 116–18, 117f; revising operating plan based on learning, 123–25, 123t

Journey Leadership Toolkit, 211; Diagnostic Worksheet for the Team Builder (developing an open partnership culture), 215; Leadership Checkup, 219–21; Worksheet for the Advocate (getting stakeholders on board), 217; Worksheet for the Convener (assuring effective meeting management), 212; Worksheet for the Networker (leveraging connections), 218; Worksheet for the Political Influencer (getting officials on board), 218; Worksheet for the Strategist (updating the strategy), 214; Worksheet for the Team Builder (managing conflict), 216; Worksheet for the Visionary (maintaining focus on achieving the overall goal), 213

Journey Management Toolkit, 197–98; Balanced Scorecard, 202, 203t; Checklist for Holding Productive Meetings, 206–7t; Communications Plan Template, 203, 204t, 205; Milestone-guided Activity Debriefing, 209; Opportunity Matrix, 200, 201t; partner feedback survey (10,000-Mile Checkup), 208; Problem Statement Worksheet, 198–99; Worksheet for Sharing Credit, 205–6

Kantor, David, 59–60

Katzenbach, Jon R., 91, 92, 98

Kickbusch, Ilona, 24

Kim, Jim Yong: on coordinating efforts, 170; on evaluation by funders, 163; on goals of partnerships, 116; on lessons learned, 152–53; MDR-TB PARTNERS project

Kim, Jim Yong *(continued)*
  and, 70, 71, 74, 79, 80, 82, 83, 152–
  53; on relations with partners, 122;
  on science of scale-up in global
  health, 168
Krug, Etienne, 139–40

Last Mile, 13, 80–83, 81f, 143–46;
  adapting strategy, 150–51; adapting
  the approach to sustain momentum, 146–51; capturing and communicating lessons learned, 152–
  54; dissolving the partnership,
  154–55; involving local stakeholders, 150; key elements, 146–55, 146f;
  meanings of, 80; transferring control and giving credit, 151–52
Last Mile Toolkit, 222; adapting and
  continuously improving intervention strategy, 225; discussion guide
  for partnership dissolution, 232;
  grantee feedback to donor, 241–
  42t; identifying and communicating lessons learned, 230–31t; involving local stakeholders, 224;
  partnership self-evaluation, 228–
  29t; recipient country feedback to
  donor, 236, 237–38t; refocusing the
  approach to surveillance, 223;
  Transferring Control Checklist,
  226; Worksheet: Developing a
  Senior Fellows Program, 235–36;
  Worksheet: Examples of Impact
  Measurement, 235; Worksheet:
  Planning a Priority Forum on a
  Specific Disease/Threat, 240–41t;
  Worksheet: Planning Investment
  in a Leadership Center, 239–40t;
  Worksheet: Providing Active
  Learning to Grantees, 238–39t;
  Worksheet for Sharing Credit,
  227–28

lead partner (governance model), 96t
leaders of partnerships, opportunities
  and challenges facing, 29–30
leadership: complementary, 79–80
  (*see also* leadership roles, complementary); importance, 127–29. *See
  also* Journey Leadership Toolkit
leadership and management skills, xii;
  supporting development of,
  167–69
leadership roles: complementary,
  127–42, 128f (*see also* leadership,
  complementary); critical external,
  137–42, 137t. *See also* team leadership roles
learning, active, 169
Lehman, Rob, 7
Lesotho, HIV/AIDS victims in, 82
Lewis, Stephen, 4, 176
Linden, Russell M., 3, 5, 59, 63, 133
local organizations, work with,
  162–63
local skills, building, 164–65
Lyman, Richard, 86
lymphatic filariasis (LF), 58–59

Mahler, Halfdan T., 86, 147
malaria, 2. *See also* Roll Back Malaria
  Partnership
management: circumstances that
  make it daunting, 109–10; discipline and flexibility in, 78–79,
  108–25, 110f. *See also* Journey Management Toolkit; leadership and
  management skills
McIntyre, Margaret H., 17
MDR-TB (multi-drug-resistant TB),
  17–19, 69
MDR-TB PARTNERS project, 17,
  69–70; First Mile, 72–76; Genesis
  of a partnership, 70–72; Jim Kim
  and, 70, 71, 74, 79, 80, 82, 83, 152–

53; Journey, 76–80; Last Mile, 80–83

measles, 73–74; vaccine, 32, 36

Mectizan, 113, 124–25

Mectizan Donation Program (MDP), 52–53, 57–59

Mectizan Expert Committee (MEC), 124

membership (of partnership): choosing the right, 73, 88–93; limiting to a manageable size, 92–93

Merck, 52–53, 57, 58, 124

Merson, Mike, 43–44, 163, 170

MINSA. See Peruvian Ministry of Health

mission statements, worksheet for developing, 183–85

multi-drug-resistant TB. See MDR-TB

Myers-Briggs Type Indicator, 63

National Highway Traffic Safety Administration (NHTSA), 39–40

National Immunization Days (NIDs), 95, 159

National Onchocerciasis Task Force, 122–23

natural disasters, 5, 7

networker (external leadership role), 139–41, 218

nongovernmental development organizations (NGDOs), 113, 115

nongovernmental organizations (NGOs), 27–28, 168

onchocerciasis (river blindness), 2, 11t, 52–53. See also African Program for Onchocerciasis Control

Onchocerciasis Control Program (OCP), 58, 113

open (organizational) culture, 59, 60, 61t

opportunities, 188. See also SWOT

opportunity matrix, 189–90

organizational agenda, 181

organizational cultures: differences in, 57–61; expectations of agency and nonagency partners, 59–61, 60t; types of, 59–61, 61t

organizational roles, 191; clarifying, 75–76, 102–5; in PARTNERS, 76, 76t; questions for determining, 191; in Roll Back Malaria Partnership, 102–3, 102t, 137

Ottesen, Eric, 57, 59, 151

Pan American Health Organization (PAHO), 147

Pandak, Carol, 123

Partners in Health (PIH), 71, 76t, 77

Partnership Against Resistant Tuberculosis: A Network for Equity and Resource Sharing (PARTNERS): First Mile, 73–76; Journey, 77–79; Last Mile, 79–83; naming of, 73; organizational roles in, 76, 76t. See also MDR-TB PARTNERS project

Partnership Pathway, 69, 70f. See also First Mile; Journey; Last Mile

partnerships. See global health partnerships

Pearson, Clarence E., 139

PEPFAR, 28

personality differences. See individuals

Peruvian Ministry of Health (MINSA), 76t, 81

planning, 13; applying discipline in, 111–14; time wasted in poor, 111. See also under Journey

policies, adapting to strengthen support for infrastructure, 164–67 policymaking phase ("scaling-up" stage), 48–49

polio, Rotary International efforts to eradicate, 157–59

polio eradication efforts in the Americas, Last Mile of, 146–48; adapting strategy, 151; shifting the approach to surveillance, 148–50

polio partnership of the Americas, 11t

political influencer (external leadership role), 138–39, 218

political will, uniting to build, 36

"political will" stage (of dealing with disease/threat), 43–45, 43t

positive attitude, 91

prevention and treatment, integration of, 21–22

priorities: forums for discussing, 171–72; sponsoring forums for leaders to reach consensus on, 169–72

problem solving, continuously engaging partners in, 119–20; communicating frequently with partners, 122–23; holding productive meetings, 120–22; principles for, 120t

program-delivery phase ("scaling-up" stage), 49–50

project planning, 78

public health, regional and national differences in views about, 5

Public Health Informatics Institute, 120

random (organizational) culture, 60, 61, 61t

real collaboration, 7, 183; defined, 7; purpose, 176–77; why it is challenging, 13. See also specific topics

research and planning, applying discipline in, 111–14

research and planning processes, principles for, 111, 112t

research phase ("scaling-up" stage), 46–47

resources, 20, 21f

"river blindness." See onchocerciasis

roads, redesigning three-lane, 44–45

road-traffic injuries, 11t; social and political systems that affect, 48–49; threshold in data and communication, 39–41

Roll Back Malaria Partnership (RBM), 2, 89, 90, 102; organizational roles in, 102–3, 102t, 137

Rosenberg, Mark L.: on David Ward, 132–33; on differences between individuals, 62–63; GRS SC and, 129–32, 138; on interplay of leadership roles, 136; on lessons from experience, 70; MDR-TB PARTNERS project and, 17–19, 71, 78, 79; on need for team builder, 134–36; as networker, 139; as team builder, 135–36; on Tony Bliss, 133; United Nations and, 138

Ross, David, 55, 73, 102, 119–20, 167

Rotary International, 157–59

roundabouts, building, 44

Rowitz, Lou, 57

Sabin, Albert, 156

Salk, Jonas, 86

"scaling-up" stage (of dealing with disease/threat), 45, 46t; policymaking phase, 48–49; program-delivery phase, 49–50; research phase, 45, 46t, 47

secretariat (governance model), 96t

"seed capital of trust," 105

shared goal, developing a, 73–74, 93–94; language/topics relating to the goal, 94–95; vision, 94 shareholder model, 88

sharing credit for successes, 118, 205–6, 227–28

Sidibé, Michel, 26, 164, 168

skills, 182; experience and technical/functional, 91; looking for individuals with needed, 90–91. *See also* leadership and management skills

smallpox, 11t, 31–32, 36; evolution of global health efforts to address, 36–37, 37f

smallpox eradication program, 143–50

Smith, Douglas K., 91, 92, 98

Smith, Ian, 28, 30, 85, 88, 105, 132

Sobel, Rochelle, 140

"social organization," 71

social responsibility, 22

Socios en Salud (SES), 71, 76t, 77

Soni, Anil, 57, 119, 173

South African AIDS Vaccine Initiative (SAAVI), 111

Special Program for Research and Training in Tropical Diseases (TDR), 53, 57, 115

stakeholder analysis: for potential individual members, 182; for potential member organizations, 180–81

stakeholder groups: defining critical, 88–91; types of partnership and, 88–91, 89t

stakeholder model, 88

Stansfield, Sally, 161–62, 166–67

STOP-TB initiative, 2

strategist (team leadership role), 133, 214

strategy worksheet, 190

strategy(ies): adapting, 150–51, 225; continuously improving, 225; examples of, 101t; shaping a big-picture, 75, 98–102

strengths, 188. *See also* SWOT

structure, selecting an appropriate (First Mile), 74–75, 95–98

surveillance efforts, 148–50, 223

sustainability, grants and, 162–63

Sweden, 44–45

SWOT (strengths, weaknesses, opportunities, and threats) analysis, 187–89

synchronous (organizational) culture, 60, 61, 61t

Taliento, Lynn, 47

Tanzania: players tackling AIDS in, 26f; Roll Back Malaria project in, 102 (*see also* Roll Back Malaria Partnership)

Task Force for Child Survival and Development, 1–2, 8f, 48, 71, 76t; First Mile, 85, 87; National Immunization Days and, 95; organizational roles in, 103–4, 104t; and representation by stakeholders, 93; strategy and, 100–102; supporting structures and, 98. *See also* Task Force for Global Health

Task Force for Global Health (Task Force), 9. *See also* Task Force for Child Survival and Development

TDR. *See* Special Program for Research and Training in Tropical Diseases

team builder, 133–36, 215, 216

team leadership roles, 129t; filling critical, 129–37

team orientation, 91

teamwork, indicators of, 182

threats, 188–89. *See also* disease/threat; SWOT

Thylefors, Bjorn, 59, 113–15, 124

tobacco, 11t

tuberculosis (TB), 2, 11t, 17–19. *See also* MDR-TB

Twum-Danso, Nana, 91

UNAIDS, 2, 49; development, 12, 44
United Nations (UN): Millennium
    Development Goals, 171–72;
    NGOs and, 27–28; organizations,
    24, 25f, 26; political correctness,
    92; Seth Berkley on, 92. *See also
    under* Global Road Safety Steering
    Committee; UNAIDS
United Nations Children's Fund
    (UNICEF), 86, 130

vaccinations, 1–2, 11t. *See also under
    specific diseases*
vaccine-preventable diseases, 2
Villeneuve, Pascal, 90–91
vision, 94
vision statements, worksheet for
    developing, 183–85
visionary (team leadership role),
    132–33, 213

Walt, Gill, 24, 26, 28
Ward, David, 132–33, 138, 140
Warnke, Paul, 145
Warren, Kenneth, 93, 94
Watson, William, 97
weaknesses, 188. *See also* SWOT
World Bank, 1
World Health Assembly (WHA),
    31–32
World Health Organization (WHO),
    76t; history, 24, 28; HIV/AIDS
    and, 43–44; smallpox and, 31–32;
    Task Force for Child Survival and,
    1; tuberculosis and, 82–83
*World Report on Road Traffic Injury
    Prevention,* 140

Yach, Derek, 166
Yip, Ray, 56, 89

Zeitz, Paul, 172
Zintl, Paul, 80–82

Text: 11/14 Adobe Garamond
Display: Gill Sans Book
Compositor: BookMatters, Berkeley
Printer and binder: Maple-Vail Book Manufacturing Group